Grace W. Weinstein

People Study People

THE STORY OF PSYCHOLOGY

E. P. Dutton   New York

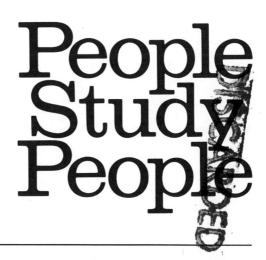

The engraving used on the jacket and chapter opening pages is a nine-teenth-century cut from *Harter's Picture Archive for Collage and Illustration*, edited by Jim Harter, and published by Dover Publications, Inc.

The author gratefully acknowledges permission to use the following copyrighted material: page 28 adaptation of Epigenetic Chart from *Childhood and Society*, by Erik H. Erikson, Copyright 1950, © 1963 by W. W. Norton & Company, Inc., and used with their permission; pages 40–41 adaptation of chart from "The Origin of Personality" by Alexander Thomas, Stella Chess, and Herbert G. Birch. Copyright © 1970 by Scientific American Inc., used by permission of W. H. Freeman and Company for Scientific American, Inc.; and page 125, chart entitled "Developmental Periods in Early and Middle Adulthood" from *The Seasons of a Man's Life* by Daniel J. Levinson, Copyright © 1978 by Daniel J. Levinson, used by permission of the author and the publisher, Alfred A. Knopf, Inc.

Library of Congress Cataloging in Publication Data

Weinstein, Grace W.   People study people.
Bibliography: p.   Includes index.
SUMMARY: Traces the development of psychology including psychoanalysis, behaviorism, humanism, and contemporary psychological research.
1. Psychology. [1. Psychology. 2. Psychiatry] I. Title.
BF139.W4   1979   150'.19   79–9996   ISBN: 0-525-36855-8

Published in the United States by E. P. Dutton, a Division of Elsevier-Dutton Publishing Company, Inc., New York
Published simultaneously in Canada by Clarke, Irwin & Company Limited, Toronto and Vancouver

Editor: Ann Troy   Designer: Patricia Lowy
Printed in the U.S.A.   First Edition   10 9 8 7 6 5 4 3 2 1

For my family, with love

CONTENTS

I exist in my dreams where e'er they go
I follow the paths that they lead me to
Although reluctant I must wake I know
   At night I am a person I don't know
   My inner feelings I often pursue
   I exist in my dreams where e'er they go
At times I go down to the world below
And sometimes I sit with the morning dew
Although reluctant I must wake I know
   Down the paths of my mind the waters flow
   To my subconscious I look for a clue
   I exist in my dreams where e'er they go
Within my slumber I have not a foe
The images shown may well be quite true
Although reluctant I must wake I know
   Happenings often are from long ago
   As dreams come to a close, my time is through,
   I exist in my dreams where e'er they go
   Although reluctant I must wake I know

         Janet Weinstein

People Study People

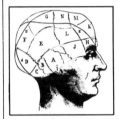

In the beginning

Psychology is a modern science but an ancient quest. People have always wondered about human behavior, about human emotions. In the absence of visible causes, the earliest men and women attributed extremes of behavior and emotion—violence, exhilaration, depression, and insanity itself—to extrahuman forces, to gods and goddesses and the powers of nature. These powers had to be placated through ritual.

The root causes of all human behavior, in fact, were eventually sought through religion, through the more-than-human. If a man was a natural leader, taking command of his tribe, it was not his doing but that of the forces that willed it to be so. If another was smarter than his neighbors, finding a better way to provide food, this too was attributable to outside forces.

The earliest religions, like those we know today, provided

1

explanations for the creation of the world and the creation of people within that world. The earliest people, in seeking answers, looked first to the power of things they could see but not necessarily understand: the sky, the sun, the animals that dominated their lives. Gradually, belief in these forces of nature shifted to belief in superhuman spiritual beings, in gods and goddesses, each of whom controlled some particular element of human nature. More gradually still, belief in these multiple representations of the unknown, these multiple explanations for human nature, shifted (for most of the world's population) to belief in a single God.

Today, after centuries of study and speculation, religion continues to play a major role in many explanations of human behavior. It's probably safe to say that it always will. Alongside religion, however, in the twentieth century, stands the scientific laboratory. Here biologists and chemists and geologists study the technical origin of life. Here psychologists examine human behavior, analyzing brain waves and perception, learning patterns and dreams. Before we look at some of the research taking place in psychological laboratories today, let's define *psychology* and look back at its origins.

Definitions

The word *psychology* stems from *psyche*, the Greek word for "soul" or "spirit," often pictured as a fragile butterfly. Legend describes Psyche as a beautiful maiden, so beautiful that Cupid, son of the goddess Venus, fell in love with her. Venus disapproved of this match between god and mortal, and Psyche was compelled to wander the world, performing tasks assigned by Venus, before winning immortality through faithfulness to her Cupid.

Today Psyche's spirit lingers. We use the word *psyche* itself to mean soul or mind, a person's inner being. The word *psychology*, stemming from *psyche*, defines the study of the

2

human mind. *Psychiatry,* a word with the same root, refers to the study of abnormal behavior. Other forms of Psyche's name appear in the words *psychic,* a person who is supposed to sense things with the mind, and *psychosomatic,* an illness originating in the mind. (Psychosomatic illnesses, by the way, are real illnesses, physical complaints tied to the psyche. A tense person, reacting to emotional stress, may develop the irritation of the stomach lining known as an ulcer.)

Although the words come from the same root, there is a difference between psychology and psychiatry. Psychology deals with the entire range of human behavior, thought, and emotion. It is a behavioral science, dealing with normal behavior as well as with abnormal, with what human beings do and feel within the range of accepted behavior and outside that range. It deals with individuals and with groups. Psychologists, with postgraduate training in psychology, work in laboratories and in clinics, in schools and in business and industry. Psychologists study the causes of behavior, conducting laboratory and clinical research, with animals and with people, into motivation and learning and memory. They treat behavioral problems, working with individuals and with groups. And they provide counseling, helping people make career and educational and personal choices.

Psychiatry, on the other hand, is a branch of medicine which concentrates on behavioral disturbances, on the moderate and severe forms of behavior which are sometimes characterized as mental or emotional illness. Psychiatrists complete the entire course of study that all physicians complete, then specialize in psychiatry. Psychiatrists use the counseling methods used by psychologists; as doctors of medicine, they can also prescribe drugs in treatment.

There is some overlap between the interests of psychology and psychiatry. There is also some overlap, some fuzziness of definition, between the "normal" and the "abnormal," between behavior which does not need treatment and behavior which does. Some behavior is clearly irrational: The "Son of Sam" murders in New York in 1977 and the axe murders of Swedish tourists on the streets of Moscow in 1978 were performed by individuals sorely in need of help. Other mental and/or emotional disturbances may be equally real but may be disturbing only to the individual: The anxiety-ridden woman who cannot function on the job and the depressed man who can no longer talk to his family both have real problems but are not threatening to society.

Psychotic individuals (*psychosis* is another word rooted in *psyche*) suffer from severely impaired mental processes; they may not be murderers—some are extremely withdrawn— but they are unable to recognize reality. Many psychotics (as many as half of those hospitalized in the United States) suffer from some form of schizophrenia, from a Greek word meaning "splitting of the mind"; schizophrenics are characterized by the fragmented nature of their thoughts and feelings. Many schizophrenics, but not all, are paranoid, sure that they are being persecuted. Schizophrenia is a form of psychosis currently thought to have a biochemical cause.

Neurotic individuals, on the other hand, may have difficulty with one aspect of life or another but are still very much in touch with reality. They go to school or work, take care of themselves, and interact with other people. They may, however, be generally anxious, with a kind of nonspecific or free-floating dread. Or they may have a phobia, a fear of a particular object, place, or sensation. If it bothers them enough, they may seek help in overcoming the neurosis. Or they may try to deal with it themselves, with more or less success. The victim of free-floating anxiety may think she is anxious because of demands at work; she may change jobs and find that she is just as anxious in the new position. The person who is afraid of heights may simply avoid them. It's generally possible, if sometimes inconvenient, to avoid heights. The person with a broad-based phobia such as claus-

4

trophobia, however, may have more difficulty sidestepping the source of his fears. Distress in closed spaces nearly precludes urban living in the last quarter of the twentieth century.

Other personality disturbances may be temporary reactions to all-too-real events. Inconsolable grief over an untimely death may produce depression and interfere with day-to-day life; such grief is normal, not neurotic, as long as it does not continue indefinitely. Overwhelming fear may produce anxiety and an inability to act, but under certain circumstances may be perfectly justified; fearlessness, in fact, would be abnormal for a kidnap victim.

Still other behavior may not bother the individual or threaten others but may be annoying or irritating to some people. The man who mutters to himself as he walks down the street and the woman who collects stray animals till her house is bulging may or may not need help, depending at least in part on the perceptions of those around them. Such people may be viewed as harmless eccentrics, entitled to their individually chosen quirks of behavior. Or they may be seen as cases, harmless or not, whose behavior should be brought into line.

The problem lies in the definition of normality. People are often considered to be behaving normally when they function well—at home, on the job, and in relationships with other people. Yet this definition, although it appears to be practical in terms of everyday life, is troublesome. For one thing, it is subjective: Who determines whether someone is functioning well? The woman who collects stray animals may be certain she is doing the right thing; her neighbors may be equally certain that her behavior, upsetting as it is to the tranquility of the neighborhood and to their property values, is over the edge. For another, it implies that conformity to the expectations of others is a virtue. We pride ourselves on individual freedom. But under this definition of normality,

5

extremes of behavior and of emotion may be considered abnormal because they make others uncomfortable.

Who are the "others" who determine normality? Some behaviors are objected to by some people while appreciated by other people. The radical leader out to change society has a band of devoted followers who believe in their cause all the more because the mass of people fail to see the light. The consumer advocate may have the support of countless "little people," while earning the enmity of those with special interests. The high-spirited youngster may liven his classmates' day with his pranks, while driving the teacher to the wall. Should the radical leader be committed to an institution because most people are disturbed by his politics? Should the consumer advocate be hushed up because powerful people object to his stance? Should the youngster be referred for therapy because the teacher finds his pranks disruptive? Or is it possible that some behavior may present a problem, to the individual or to others, without being a mental disorder in need of treatment?

If normality, in other words, is defined in a way that implies conformity, then a great many people are abnormal: people who talk to themselves or dress in unconventional ways or collect stray animals; people who react emotionally to injustice; people who are depressed or anxious or fearful; people who march, in whatever way, to the beat of a different drummer. If normality is defined in terms of average behavior, furthermore, then cultural differences do not count. And we know that different cultures have different expectations about normal behavior.

Anthropologists have demonstrated that some cultures value aggression, while others are peace-loving; some encourage competition, while others stress cooperation; some have designated roles for men and women that are very different from the designated roles in neighboring tribes or nations. Men may be the hunters and food gatherers—or the storytellers, the keepers of tradition. Women may be passive, deferring to the wishes of men, while nurturing the children—or they may be the hunters, the source of material wealth. Children may be expected to be seen and not heard—or to be noisy and aggressive, full participants in family life.

The differences may be seen in field studies with primitive tribes. They may also be seen among modern industrialized nations. And they are evident within the United States in groups stemming from different cultures. When different cultures clash, one or the other may be called abnormal. In one study, for instance, nurses were asked whether or not they were good nurses. While eleven out of twelve Americans, reflecting the American belief that self-confidence is a virtue, proclaimed their own competence, those of Norwegian background modestly refused to say. Is modesty normal or abnormal? Is self-confidence?

Normality, in short, is frequently defined by expectations. You can determine this yourself. Ask someone to observe the strange behavior of a man waiting at a bus stop. The man may be doing nothing more unusual than fidgeting while he waits for an overdue bus. But your friend, prompted to look for something strange, may see what he looks for. "Yes," he may say, "that man seems awfully nervous; maybe he's paranoid, thinks someone is chasing him."

We see what we expect to see. So do professionals in the field of mental health. This was made painfully clear in 1972 when David Rosenhan, a Stanford University psychologist, had himself and several other people admitted to mental institutions. The "patients" each claimed that they heard voices. In every other respect they told the truth; they recounted their own life stories and behaved in their own accustomed ways. Yet no staff member, in these reputable institutions, ever discovered the charade. No psychiatrist or psychologist, social worker or nurse ever suspected the truth, even when the "patients" began openly interviewing other patients, taking notes, and ignoring prescribed medication. Expectations proved so strong, in fact, that the note taking was interpreted as pathological behavior, confirmation of mental illness. The "patients" were eventually released, diagnosed as "schizophrenics in remission"—sick people, in other words, temporarily free from symptoms.

Expectations also work the other way. In a later experiment, Rosenhan told the staff of a major institution that a number of people would seek admission under false pretenses; just as he had done earlier, they would claim to be disturbed when they were in fact normal. Although there actually were no such "patients," the staff, primed to expect them, found quite a few. The line between normal behavior and abnormal behavior is still fuzzy. Human behavior, in the twentieth century, may be just as much a mystery as it has always been.

Myths and legends

Early peoples, isolated in sparsely populated settlements, did not know about cultural differences or abnormal psychology or expectations of normality. But they were keenly aware of human behavior. They tried to explain that behavior within the framework of the world, as they understood the world. In doing so, they often turned to supernatural explanations. Much was attributed to the extraordinary power of nature. The power of the sun, the strength of the wind, the force of lightning were invoked to explain the behavior of people. Much was also attributed to beings who were larger than life, to gods and heroes who set the pattern for mankind. Myths relate how things came to be: Mankind possesses fire because Prometheus gave it as a gift. A certain tribe lives by fishing because a legendary supernatural being taught the first tribesman to catch and cook fish. And so on, across the world, across barriers of history and language and culture.

Every group has its tales, its myths and legends. We still, today, have fairy tales. And fairy tales, according to psychologist Bruno Bettelheim, are far more than simple stories told to amuse the young: They are symbolic interpretations of the inner problems of human beings and solutions to those problems. The young child sees the giant in "Jack and the Beanstalk" as symbolic of adults, often looming large and frightening, but possible to outwit through cunning. The story of Cinderella, in turn, represents sibling rivalry, the child's intense feeling that his parents favor his brothers and sisters but that he will, because of his superiority, eventually win out.

You know these stories, of Jack and of Cinderella, of Snow White and of Sleeping Beauty. But do you know the stories of Narcissus and of Oedipus? The myths which speak across the centuries, in literature and in theatre and in psychology, the ones which show up again and again in fairy tales, are the myths of the ancient Greeks. These myths also symbolize inner conflicts and their solution. But they go further, invoking superhuman heroes and divine intervention. Volumes have been devoted to recounting Greek myths; there are far too many to retell here. But it's worth a brief look at a couple of the myths, the ones which have been significant in contemporary psychological thought.

Narcissus, for example, was a beautiful young man who, upon seeing his reflection in a spring, fell in love with his own beauty. He was so entranced, according to one version of the legend, that he remained fixed by the spring, gazing at his own image, until he died. His name has similarly become fixed: Anyone entranced with his own self, wound up in his own beauty or intellect or fascination, is called narcissistic. In a psychological sense, every young child goes through a narcissistic phase, a period in which he feels that he is the center of the universe. But it is necessary to mature, to outgrow this phase. The individual who remains fixed at this stage, as Narcissus remained fixed by the spring, is unable to relate to other people, to step outside himself sufficiently to form healthy relationships. A narcissistic person is the ultimately selfish—and ultimately lonely—individual.

Oedipus, whose legend is extraordinarily important in the work of Sigmund Freud, was abandoned in infancy by his royal parents in order to forestall a prophecy which warned that he would grow up to murder his father and marry his mother. Prophecies, however, are not so easily undone. Rescued by a shepherd, the infant Oedipus was brought up as the son of a neighboring ruler. As a young man, warned of the prophecy and fearful that he would harm his parents, Oedipus left their kingdom. In his travels, still ignorant of his real parentage, he quarreled with an elderly stranger. In the ensuing fight, Oedipus killed the stranger. He did not know, as you have guessed, that the man he killed was his natural father and that he had carried out the first portion of the prophecy. Later, after helping the people of the city of Thebes, Oedipus, still all unknowing, was rewarded with the hand of their widowed queen in marriage. That queen, of course, was his mother. The classic Greek tale ends with Oedipus, at last aware of what he has done, blinding himself in retribution.

In fulfilling the prophecy, Oedipus lent his name to Freud's description of the internal conflict felt by every small child: the wish to dispossess the parent of the same sex and possess the parent of the opposite sex. This, like narcissism, is a stage that Freud said must be worked through in the normal development of every child.

The history of psychology

Throughout early history, including the period of the Greek myths, most human beings viewed mental disorders as a reflection of the anger of the gods: Oedipus went mad and blinded himself when he displeased the gods by his unnatural acts. But the myths are very ancient. By the time of Hippocrates, the founder of modern medicine, in about the fourth century B.C., some people rejected this explanation and emphasized the role of natural causes. Hippocrates himself referred to bodily types; he believed that there were four basic temperaments, or "humors," based on the relative dominance of blood, black bile, yellow bile, or phlegm. He attributed mental illness to physical causes.

Some later psychologists, on into the twentieth century, have followed Hippocrates' lead by attempting to relate personality types to physical characteristics. You may have heard of the work of W. H. Sheldon, who identified the basic body-personality types as ectomorph, endomorph, and mesomorph. The ectomorph, lean and slender, is supposed to be intellectual, sensitive, and happy to be alone. The endomorph, round and soft, loves food, comfort, and sociability. The mesomorph, strong and athletic, is energetic and aggressive. Neither Hippocrates nor Sheldon has much contemporary support. But there may well be some relationship between the physical and the psychological; current research is concentrating on biochemistry in an attempt to find the connection.

The scientific thought which flourished at the time of Hippocrates lasted only a few hundred years. Then humanity sank once again into primitive modes of thought, primitive explanations for behavior. Throughout medieval times, mental illness was explained by, if not the anger of God, then the intervention of Satan; mentally ill people were thought to be witches, possessed by demons. It was not until the seventeenth and eighteenth centuries that scientific thought re-emerged. And it was not until the eighteenth and nineteenth centuries that mentally ill people began to receive humane treatment.

Even in this period, however, psychology was not quite a science. Until the late nineteenth century, psychology was part of philosophy. Philosophers, not psychologists, considered man's behavior and sought explanations for that behavior. Philosophers, not psychologists, considered questions of consciousness, of thought, of temperament. Philosophers analyzed the emotions, looked at motivation, described intellectual functioning. Philosophers were concerned with the place of human beings in the universe, a place lower than God's but higher than the animals'.

Psychology became a separate discipline in the late nineteenth century, when Francis Galton developed the first scientifically based psychological tests. Galton, a follower of Darwin, was a biologist who was interested in the inheritance of individual differences and similarities. Differences in intellectual functioning could be determined, he thought, through differences in physical process. At his laboratory in London, therefore, he measured differences in the discrimination of stimuli, in the way in which different people sense stimulation through sight and sound and touch. He measured reaction times, the speed with which different people react to different stimuli. And, in a significant contribution to later psychology, he developed statistical means to record his results.

Galton's tests dealt with simple sensory reactions and motor functions. By the first decade of the twentieth century, Alfred Binet, at the request of French educational authorities, had developed a direct test for intelligence. The test, based on mental abilities at a given age, was a forerunner of modern intelligence tests. The intelligence quotient (IQ), or measure of intelligence as a ratio between mental age and chronological age, is based on Binet's work.

By the time of World War I, the theory of testing had been accepted. Men drafted into the U.S. Army were given a battery of psychological tests to determine what they could and could not do. In the same years, psychological researchers were busy in many other areas as well, particularly in trying to understand the reasons for human behavior.

In recent years, psychology has grown; it has spread beyond the laboratory and the therapist's office, into the classroom and the factory and the prison and the clinic. The understanding gained through psychology is applied in diverse ways: vocational counseling, product advertising, rehabilitation, opinion polling, test design, and market research are just a few. Psychologists deal with real problems of real people. But they do so according to different theoretical positions developed through the years of seeking causes for human behavior. The significant positions include psychoanalysis, based on the work of Sigmund Freud; behaviorism; the cognitive theories of Jean Piaget; and humanism. These theoretical positions, and their applications to human problems and concerns, make up the rest of this book.

PART II

Psychoanalysis: Psychology on the Couch

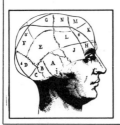

Sigmund Freud:
A theory
of the unconscious

Modern psychology began on the famous couch of the Viennese doctor Sigmund Freud. Freud did not invent psychology. But he did invent a theory of personality which recognized for the first time the workings of the unconscious mind, the power of instinctual drives, and the impact of early childhood experiences. He developed psychoanalysis. In doing so, his name became inextricably linked with psychology. You've heard his name, whether or not you know much about his work. And you've been influenced, directly or indirectly, by his discoveries.

Who was Sigmund Freud?
It helps, in understanding the theories of any great mind, to understand something of the origins of that mind. Freud,

like any human being, was stamped by the time and place in which he lived. He was influenced by his family and in turn influenced others. He was also, indisputably, a genius.

Freud was born in 1856, the oldest child and first son of the seven children born to Jakob and Amalie Freud. There were also two grown half brothers, children of Jakob Freud's earlier marriage; one of the half brothers had a son a year older than Sigmund. This older nephew was a childhood companion.

Although Freud was born in Moravia, now part of Czecho-slovakia, the family moved to Vienna when he was three. He lived in Vienna until the Nazi invasion in 1938 forced him into exile in England, where he died a year later, at the age of eighty-three. Freud was stamped by Vienna, a sophis-ticated and cultured city in which, nonetheless, opportu-nities for Jews were severely limited. Freud's early dreams of becoming a general or a minister of state were thwarted by this reality, and he turned his attention to medicine. His decision to attend medical school, however, grew out of his interest in pure research; he did not particularly want to work with patients. He opened a medical practice in neurol-ogy, eventually, only in order to earn enough money so that he could marry.

That medical practice, in which he dealt with men and women in whom no physical cause could be found for physi-cal symptoms, led directly to the development of psychoanalysis. Other doctors had previously used a combi-nation of hypnosis and what they called a "talking-out" method, in which patients were encouraged to talk freely about what was bothering them. Freud discovered that hyp-nosis was not necessary. Talking-out alone, the free associa-tion of ideas, enabled many patients to reach the root of their problems. The method, as well as the theory, is called psychoanalysis; the term was invented by Freud.

A *theory of personality development*

Freud was by training a scientist and a physician. It was only natural, therefore, that he would see the roots of personality in biology. Instincts, he claimed, are the dominant force behind human behavior. Of the instincts, the sexual instinct, expressed through the libido, is the most important.

This theory, however, is a developmental theory. Personality, according to Freud, is not established from birth. Instead, it progresses through certain stages. The normal personality, that is, progresses through each stage to maturity. The neurotic personality, personified by the troubled people who consulted Freud as a specialist in nervous disorders, had, he suspected, either "fixated" at an immature developmental stage, or had been so traumatized by the events of one stage that further normal development was impossible.

Development is lifelong. But the crucial period, the most vital in terms of personality formation, lies in the first five years of life. Freud's sequence for these years included oral, anal, and phallic stages.

The oral stage, the very first, centers around the infant's drive for satisfaction through the mouth. The degree of satisfaction and of frustration the infant experiences at this stage influences later personality development. The frustrated infant may become an adult with an "oral" character structure, an adult who is preoccupied with food . . . or who is biting and sarcastic . . . or dependent on others . . . or greedy and acquisitive, seeking to acquire things that substitute (unconsciously, of course) for the mother love expressed in infancy through food. The person tied to gratification through oral means may also, if the longing for food is repressed, be the person who chews gum, smokes, or drinks.

The anal period, which follows in the second year, has a single all-important focal point: toilet training. Parental attitudes toward control over bodily functions in general, and methods of training in particular, have a major impact, according to Freud, on the child's developing personality. Overly strict training may result in a compulsive, obstinate, retentive, meticulously neat individual. Overly strict training may also, if the individual reacts strongly, produce the opposite result: a person who relishes giving things away. Sometimes, in a person with anal characteristics, a characteristic pattern of strictly controlled behavior may be punctuated by explosive outbursts.

The phallic stage, which rounds out the first five years, is marked by the child's identification with the parents and assumption of male or female characteristics. It is also marked by a beginning awareness of sexual identity, so that the young boy, seeing that girls are different, suffers from castration anxiety. The young girl, meanwhile, seeing that boys are different, unconsciously feels penis envy. These anxieties are part of what Freud called the Oedipus complex.

The Oedipus complex, taken as a whole, provides a vivid example of Freud's thinking about the importance of the sexual instinct and about the necessary sequence of normal development. Freud made famous the ancient Greek play in which Oedipus, all unknowing, kills his father and marries his mother, by claiming that the wish to do just this is present in every boy between the ages of three and five. Freud used the Oedipus complex, in part, to support his theory that the sexual instinct begins in early childhood— and not, as his contemporaries claimed, with the onset of puberty.

In Freudian terms, it is normal for every young boy to want his mother for himself; it is also normal for him to want his father out of the way. But these feelings should be worked through in the normal course of development. If they are not, the adult, with excessively strong ties to his mother, may be unable to function well as a spouse or as a parent. Freud devoted a great deal of energy to working out his theory of the Oedipus complex, a theory which, in its pure form, applies only to males. The parallel, however, sometimes called the Electra complex, finds the young girl developing an attachment to her father while rejecting her mother.

The Oedipus complex, in both its male and female forms, reflects the turbulent feelings young children have about their parents while they are struggling to establish their own independent identity. It also contains the seeds of sibling rivalry, as small children compete with each other for parental love. Or, as Freud put it in his classic work, *A General Introduction to Psychoanalysis,* "When other children appear, the Oedipus complex expands and becomes a family complex." Most important, perhaps, is Freud's realization, although he did not work directly with children, that children have complicated feelings and emotions.

Young children, of course, do not label these feelings; nor are they, in fact, aware of them. Even later in life, mature men and women may be unaware that they ever harbored these feelings; if aware, they may repress the idea, hide it below the surface of the conscious mind. Once outgrown, once hidden, the feelings do not present a problem—unless some unsettling event triggers recognition. Her husband's heart attack, for example, prompted one woman to reexamine her feelings about her father. In her dreams, Martha Weinman Lear wrote not long ago, "The image of my husband shifts and merges sometimes with the image of my dead father. The walls of a house are crumbling. It is both my present house and the house of my childhood. . . ."

Freud would not have been surprised. Oedipal feelings are strong; they can resurface even in well-adjusted adults. Through psychoanalysis of his own patients, in fact, Freud became increasingly convinced of the long-lasting impact of childhood feelings. It was also through analysis, of his patients and of himself, that he arrived at his theory of the unconscious mind. This theory is the cornerstone of Freud's legacy, a legacy that is with us still.

The Id, the Ego, and the Superego

The unconscious, according to Freud, constitutes the largest portion of the mind, a portion which contains instincts and impulses we can rarely identify. But the unconscious is not all of a piece. It contains separate and distinct elements, identified as the id, the ego, and the superego. These separate elements, which should work together smoothly, often come into conflict. When that conflict is not resolved, neurotic symptoms may result.

The id, completely submerged in the unconscious, is the portion of the personality that demands pleasure, the immediate gratification of all desires. It is the seat of the instincts, out of touch with the real world. The id is not subject to rational thought, although it can be controlled by the ego. The id, a source of primitive energy which never changes or matures, represents the "pleasure principle." It has been called the "spoiled child of the personality." It can be held responsible for impulsive unreasoned acts.

The ego, a word sometimes used to mean the "self," has a distinct Freudian meaning as the "reality principle" of the mind. It is the ego, accommodating the demands of the id to the reality of the outside world, that makes rational behavior possible. The ego gradually matures, as a child learns that not all instincts can be immediately fulfilled; the first lesson takes place shortly after birth, when the crying infant must sometimes wait for food. The ego ultimately takes charge and acts, in the well-adjusted individual, as the executive branch of the personality, the organizer of behavior.

The superego, the third branch of the personality, may be

called the conscience. It develops as the young child internalizes parental values, making them his own. The superego functions as a restraint, as a built-in personalized moral code which reflects the morals of the family and of society.

If you see something you like but can't afford—an expensive piece of jewelry, for instance, or a gadget-laden multibladed camping knife—your id might urge you to pocket it; your ego might warn that you are likely to be caught; and your superego might restrain you because theft, in itself, is wrong. The superego, however, has such high standards that any transgression, even if only a passing thought never put into action, is punished. The punishment may take the form of uncomfortable feelings of guilt. Or it may, in extreme cases, take the form of the physical symptoms Freud saw in his neurotic patients. Freud traced one woman's illness, for example, to her romantic interest in her brother-in-law, an interest she had not admitted to herself, but which her superego saw and punished.

Ego defenses
Impulses which run counter to the reality principle of the ego provoke anxiety. Anxiety can, of course, be firmly rooted in the real world; it is not only normal but quite sensible to be anxious about a real and present danger. But anxiety may also be internal, rooted in an unconscious warning that the primitive instincts of the id may take over. Such anxiety may be general, a kind of pervasive uneasiness. Such anxiety may also be specific, related to a particular ego-defying impulse, such as the urge to steal. Again, however, the individual is rarely aware of the real source of internal anxiety, even when the anxiety is so severe that it has become a full-fledged phobia. A person deathly afraid of high places may rationalize that fear, pointing to the built-in danger of lean-

ing over a cliff . . . but that person may unconsciously be fearful of an unrecognized impulse to inflict self-punishment by jumping.

The ego must, however, defend itself against excessive anxiety. It does so through defense mechanisms, behavior which is adopted automatically, without conscious thought, when the ego senses a threat. After a fight with a friend you may, for example, displace anger, by blowing up at your mother. You may rationalize a poor test grade, and project the blame for your failure onto your teacher. Such ego defenses are not all bad. Defense mechanisms, occasionally adopted, are essential if human beings are to function. But when they are used excessively, they may lead to neurotic behavior.

Freud identified several varieties of defense mechanisms. Among them are repression, regression, and sublimation.

Repression occurs when the ego buries the anxiety-provoking material, when memory "blocks" traumatic ideas or impulses. This may, in a more complete form, result in denial. Some people may repress or deny sexual instincts. Others, in a form of repression called reversal, may convert one drive to its opposite: The person who acts aggressively independent may actually be masking feelings of dependency or a real need for other people. The school clown, who appears to have no qualms about looking foolish, may actually be painfully shy, lacking confidence in his ability to secure attention except through outrageous behavior.

Regression takes place when events at a particular developmental stage are so troublesome that an individual retreats to the security and comfort of an earlier stage. A small child may retreat to babyhood, to enjoying a bottle and forgetting that toilet training ever took place, when a new brother or sister joins the family. Such a regression is usually temporary.

Sublimation occurs when instinctive drives for personal gratification give way to socially acceptable goals and behavior. The sexual energy of the libido may find expression, for example, in artistic creativity. Aggressive instincts may be sublimated by a strongly competitive business drive. You may expend a lot of energy on sports or hobbies.

Psychoanalytic theory and therapy

Freud traced the specific dynamics of defense mechanisms just as he traced the overall workings of the unconscious mind, through past experience. He approached past experience through free association and the interpretation of dreams. He used both methods in developing his theory of personality. And he used them in providing treatment.

Free association is the Freudian psychoanalytic technique. It relies on the patient, with minimal contribution from the analyst, to talk and, in talking, make connections between significant events. The significance may be symbolic and require interpretation, but much of the work is left to the patient. Traditionally, in fact, the patient does not even see the analyst, who sits behind the head of the analytic couch. Freud began this particular tradition because, as he put it, "I cannot put up with being stared at by other people for eight hours a day. . . ."

People frequently recount their dreams in the process of free association, and the interpretation of dreams is particularly important in understanding Freud. Throughout history, philosophers have been interested in dreams. But Freud, who viewed dreams as the workings of the unconscious mind, workings in which frustrations and motivations and ego defenses can be clearly seen, brought the interpretation of dreams into the science of psychoanalysis. His major work on the subject, *The Interpretation of Dreams*, in which he analyzed his own dreams as well as those of his patients (an unusual step, because it revealed his own unconscious mind to the world), was published in 1900.

Conflicts between the id and the ego, conflicts censored by the conscious mind, can come to the surface during dreams. Then, when the conscious mind has relaxed its guard, unfulfilled wishes can be expressed. But such wishes, even in dreams, may be disguised or hidden; the message may be condensed, and the defenses set up by the ego may cause the underlying conflict to be portrayed in symbolic form. Thus, although you may be able to interpret some of your own dreams, many dreams, especially those which reflect severe conflict, may be too complicated. According to Freud, interpreting such dreams requires the help of a trained analyst.

In line with Freud's emphasis of the sexual instinct, he believed that many dreams express unfulfilled sexual wishes. He developed whole categories of symbols which he held to represent the sexual: Snakes, trees, poles, knives, and guns are among the symbols said to represent the male; houses, churches, rooms, and containers of all kinds represent the female. Such symbols, later psychologists have held, may indeed represent the sexual in particular dreams of particular people—but they may also have other meanings in other dreams, depending on the person and the context. Not all dreams, in any case, are a reflection of unrestrained libido. Some, including those in children, may be wish fulfillment tied to actual experience. An example is a small boy's dream of being on top of a mountain, an actual mountain he had dearly wanted to climb but could not manage. Another example is a teenager's dream of resounding applause after a performance in a school play, a play that has yet to be performed.

Hidden motivations may also show up in inadvertent errors, in accidents of behavior, forgetfulness, and so-called "slips of the tongue," or "Freudian slips." Freud maintained, in fact, that there is no such thing as an accident; errors result from inner conflict and "mistakes have a meaning." Finding the meanings is somewhat like tracing the clues in a detective story. He cites many examples: The woman who forgets an acquaintance's married name disapproves of the marriage; the man who loses a pencil given him by his brother-in-law does so after a quarrel with the brother-in-law; the person who forgets an appointment never wanted to keep it. Think about it the next time you dial one friend's telephone number when you really meant to call another.

In verbal "mistakes," one word may be substituted for another at the suggestion of the unconscious: A hard-drinking and hard-fighting general is called "bottle-scarred" instead of "battle-scarred"; a crown prince becomes a "clown prince." Or a word may change the consciously intended meaning to one more in line with the unconscious: A young woman told Freud that her husband did not need a special medically advised diet; "he can eat and drink," she said, "what *I* want."

The unconscious, in short, has its secrets . . . but an observer trained in Freudian psychoanalytic techniques can break the code.

Successors to Freud

Freud's revolutionary notions of the power of the unconscious mind have come to us through his own extensive writings and through a long line of dedicated followers. Because Freud invented psychoanalysis, early practitioners followed his theory and his technique virtually to the letter. It didn't take long, however, before there was dissension in the ranks. Even such a seemingly simple question as how long psychoanalysis should last (Months? Years?) or the length of the analytic hour (fifty-five minutes, as Freud himself practiced? Fifty minutes, as contemporary analysts do? Variable time, depending on the patient?) provoked intense discussion.

The quarrels, however, were much like those within a family, with an intensity of feeling comparable in many ways to sibling rivalry. Freud himself could be intensely competitive, refusing to speak with or ever forgive those who differed with him. But as the "family" grew each year, as more people became involved in the psychoanalytic movement, differences were bound to occur. Inevitably, some of the differences were serious, involving basic theory as well as details of application. Some of Freud's original followers broke away. Others never parted company with orthodox Freudian thought but extended his theories into new areas.

There are many men and women who are important in the history of psychoanalysis after Freud; some adhered strictly to his theories, while others took a fork in the road and a separate path. This book can just touch on a few of the important people and ideas before turning to the impact of Freud and psychoanalysis on our own lives.

Alfred Adler, an early associate of Freud's, later broke away and founded a school within the psychoanalytic movement. The school, called "individual psychology" because Adler emphasized the unity of the individual personality, focused on the conscious processes of the mind instead of the unconscious. Adler, furthermore, de-emphasized the sexual instinct and the libido as motivating elements in human behavior. The dominant goal in personality formation, he held, was a striving for superiority, a striving rooted in every child's feeling of inferiority. Adler, in fact, coined the term *inferiority complex*.

Carl Gustav Jung, a Swiss psychiatrist, was another early associate of Freud's who broke away and founded his own

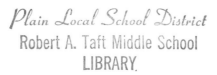

school. Jung differed from Freud in several important ways. He rejected sexuality as a primary motivating force and defined libido as the will to live. He described the unconscious as both individual and collective, the collective portion being a kind of common human ancestry. And he held that it was more important to work through current conflicts than to dwell on conflicts that had taken place in childhood. He held, in fact, that there can be a neurotic desire to return to the past as a way of avoiding the present. Jung classified personality types, including the now famous introvert and extrovert. He was concerned with religion and with mysticism, and in the 1930s was accused of supporting Naziism.

Two of the most important Freudians, who have continued and expanded Freud's concepts, are Anna Freud and Erik. H. Erikson.

Anna Freud, youngest child of and spiritual heir to Sigmund Freud, has become famous for the analysis of children. Although her father developed significant ideas about the psychology of children, he did so through the memories of his adult patients. He never worked directly with children. Anna Freud brought the experiences of a nursery-school teacher, her first career, to the analysis of children. She made her name in England, during and after World War II, in her work with young children separated from their parents by the war. These normal children, who seemed to regress when separated from their parents, indicated that environmental influences had to be considered alongside biological instincts in the development of personality. Anna Freud's strong concern for the environmental influence, for the ways in which children are treated by the family and by society, comes through in her recent book, *Beyond the Best Interests of the Child*. In this book, written with Joseph Goldstein of the Yale University Law School and Albert J. Solnit of the Yale University Child Study Center, an awareness of children's emotional needs is applied to the framework of laws dealing with the placement of children: in adoption, foster care, and custody.

Erik H. Erikson, an artist as a young man, was trained by Anna Freud as a child analyst. By 1933, however, he had settled in Boston, away from the tight-knit circle of Freud's followers in Vienna. Erikson, still in direct line with Freud's thinking, has expanded orthodox Freudian concepts. He has made several distinctive contributions: He was among the first to recognize that development is lifelong, throughout the life cycle. He has stressed the importance of identity formation, and has acknowledged that the "identity crisis" may be the most important conflict in adolescence. And, as an outgrowth of his belief in the strength of the ego as contrasted to the primitive instincts of the id, Erikson has emphasized sociocultural influences on personality.

Erikson has postulated "eight ages of man," eight stages in personality formation. In each of the eight stages, from infancy through old age, there is a conflict involving individual identity. Each stage builds on the stage before (see chart on page 28). Each stage has either a positive or a negative outcome. At the outset, for instance, there is a conflict between trust and mistrust. If physical needs are satisfied, infants learn to trust people and to depend on them; if those needs are not met, the seeds of mistrust are sown.

The school-age child, in stage 4, develops either a sense of self-confidence or a sense of inferiority. The adolescent in stage 5, which Erikson calls Identity vs. Role Confusion, is struggling to find an identity. And young adults in stage 6, having established an identity, a sense of self, are ready to move on to intimate relationships with other people. Adults in middle years face either continued creativity or stagnation, while those toward the end of life must resolve the conflict between ego integrity, the acceptance of the inevitable end of life, and despair. The struggle for growth, according to Erikson, continues throughout life.

Erik H. Erikson's "Eight Ages of Man"
(Adapted from *Childhood and Society* by Erik H. Erikson)

CONFLICT	APPROXIMATE AGE		POSITIVE OUTCOME OF THE CONFLICT
1 Basic trust vs. Mistrust	CHILDHOOD	First year	Confidence in other people and in oneself.
2 Autonomy vs. Shame and Doubt		Second to third year	Self-control leading to a lasting sense of good will and pride.
3 Initiative vs. Guilt		Third to fifth year	Moral responsibility developed through cooperative action and purposeful learning.
4 Industry vs. Inferiority		Sixth year to puberty	Competence born out of mastery of skills and tasks.
5 Identity vs. Role Confusion	ADOLESCENCE AND YOUNG ADULTHOOD	Adolescence	A sense of one's self and one's role in life, an "identity."
6 Intimacy vs. Isolation		Early adulthood	A readiness for intimacy with another person, for commitment and mature love.
7 Generativity vs. Stagnation	MATURITY	Middle age	Productivity and creativity, through work and through establishing and guiding the next generation.
8 Ego integrity vs. Despair		Later adulthood	Confidence that one's life has been meaningful and that death therefore need not be feared.

Many other people and ideas have been important in the psychoanalytic movement. Yet, although orthodox Freudian theory has been discredited in some quarters as other movements in psychology have become increasingly important, Freud's thought has influenced and continues to influence our lives.

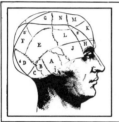 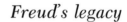

Freud's legacy

Psychoanalysis began with Freud's diagnosis of neurotic adults. The theory built on that diagnostic foundation, a theory of the unconscious mind, has spread into almost every area of life. The jargon derived from that theory, a jargon which speaks of motivations and conflicts and defense mechanisms, has infiltrated everyday speech.

Look around and you will see the wide-ranging influence of Freudian theory. It shows up in literature, in novels, and in plays. Fictional heroes are often motivated by instinctual yearnings. A mother and daughter, for instance, on the stage or screen, may fight over something trivial; the audience knows they are really expressing their rivalry over Dad. And it shows up in marketing, in the selling of goods and services. Advertisements for high-speed cars appeal to the instinct for power. Travel folders picture vacations that will satisfy the pleasure principle. Cigarette commercials have been described as glorified oral eroticism.

Freud's legacy is very much with us today. It is present, despite many competing mental-health theories and techniques, in orthodox psychoanalytic practice. It has spilled over, via projective testing, into schools and business offices. It has left a lingering mark on the nursery, in its applications to child rearing. And it has affected, in ways Freud never could have anticipated, the development of feminism.

Treatment.
The purest application of Freud's theories and practices is to be found on the analytic couch he introduced. Here, facing away from the often silent analyst, thousands of patients (or *analysands*) try to understand their inner selves. Here the same patients recount thoughts and dreams, seeking solution of adult problems through insight into childhood conflicts. The recounting is done through free association, as the patient talks on about whatever comes to mind. The analyst seldom interrupts or comments; instead, as one analyst has put it, he acts as a mirror in which the patient can see himself.

Psychoanalysts, unlike some other contemporary therapists, believe that it is impossible to resolve neuroses without getting at their roots; treating the symptoms of behavior is not enough. Psychoanalysts generally do not treat the severe personality disorders known as psychoses. They do treat people who are functioning in the world but feel they are functioning with difficulty, subject to anxiety or dependency or inadequacy of one sort or another. Many such people feel that psychoanalysis has been of real help.

But critics observe that analysts carefully select the problems they will analyze, and that this "analyzability," or likelihood of success, renders objective judgment of results impossible. Critics also suggest that analyzability may

31

occasionally create a neurosis out of normal human behavior. If it is easy to treat a minor problem, the analyst may be tempted to do so—and treatment itself, these critics suggest, labels the treated behavior as neurotic. It must be assumed, however, that most people who seek psychoanalytic help do so because they need that help in order to function to their own satisfaction.

In the analytic view, the roots of adult problems (however those problems are defined) always and inevitably lie in repressed childhood conflict. When an adult man or woman is having marital difficulties, the analyst may look to unresolved conflict with the parent of the opposite sex. When a businessman is having trouble with his supervisor, or a ballplayer is rebelling against the authority of the team manager, the analyst may help the person face the strained relationship with his father which existed throughout his childhood. The heart of it all in almost every case is the Oedipal conflict. Freudian analysts, true to Freud, see almost all human behavior in sexual terms.

Because of this insistence on the childhood origin of adult problems, Freudian analysts also, as a rule, treat the individual alone. Although some work with both husband and wife in a marital conflict, some work with the family unit, and some work with unrelated groups, many psychoanalysts treat only the primary patient. That primary patient is not necessarily the family member with the most problems, but the one who asks for help, the one considered most likely to benefit from analysis. The analyst's view of the situation may be limited, however, to what the patient chooses to reveal.

Freudian analysts, again true to Freud, believe that transference is a necessary step in analysis. The patient, in other words, transfers the intense emotions of those childhood conflicts to the person of the analyst. The love-hate relationship which develops between analyst and analysand mirrors the love-hate relationship between parent and child.

Analysis of the later relationship provides some insight into the earlier one.

Because the patient must, by himself and without much help from the analyst, work through years of life history to get at the unconscious root of problems, analysis takes a very long time. Although Freud completed some of his analyses in a matter of months, contemporary analyses often go on for years. Analysis, therefore, can cost a great deal. But it must cost a great deal relative to patient income, according to Freudians, if it is to be successful. In fact, a patient's reluctance to pay such fees is believed to indicate resistance to treatment. Similar interpretations are applied to the patient's attitude toward the fifty-minute hour. In an insider's joke, quoted by Martin Gross in *The Psychological Society,* the patient can't win. If he comes early for his sessions, he is displaying anxiety; if he is late, he is offering resistance; if he is always on time, he is compulsive.

Testing

Projective tests are also an outgrowth of Freudian theory. There are a number of such tests, all designed to elicit underlying emotions, to give the tester insight into your unconscious. They do so, and are called projective tests, because the person being tested projects his or her own emotions and feelings and responses onto situations in words or pictures which have no meaning of their own. Two of the better known of these tests are the Rorschach test and the thematic apperception test.

In the Rorschach test, the familiar inkblots, the tester presents the subject with a series of ten cards, one at a time. The tester gives no advice or instructions; he simply requests that you, the subject, tell him what you see. He then keeps track of everything you say (do you talk, or ponder in silence?) and do (do you turn the card around?). And he makes special note of the elements of the card which are

33

referred to in your response. These elements include whether you see one large figure in a blot or many small ones; the location of what you see; whether form or color seems to be most important; and the content, whether ordinary or imaginative. What you see and how you describe it is supposed to indicate your overall personality as well as any neurotic traits.

The thematic apperception test (TAT) is also based on the interpretation of pictures. In this case, the pictures are not shapeless and blurry inkblots, but people, shown in situations requiring interpretation. The person being tested is asked to provide that interpretation, as imaginatively as possible. You may, for instance, be shown a picture of a young man staring into space. The tester asks, "What is happening in this picture? What led up to this situation? What do you think will happen later?" You could respond with a description of the picture: a young man staring into space. You could attribute thoughts to him, or interpret his expression. You could weave an entire story about his life and career, his thoughts and feelings. What you say about the picture, and about all the pictures in the TAT series, is supposed to tell the tester about your own plans and goals, emotions and attitudes.

Projective tests are sometimes used in schools, where guidance counselors or psychological study teams employ them to construct a "personality profile" of students. They are also sometimes utilized in business, for job placement or job advancement. Some seventy police departments in the state of New Jersey alone, for instance, use psychological tests to screen applicants; the tests are supposed to weed out bigots, liars, and seekers after violence.

But not everyone is comfortable with psychological testing imposed on students or job seekers. There is some question, for one thing, about the objectivity of the tests themselves.

And there is uneasiness in some circles about the interpretation of the results.

The tests themselves, many critics observe, are not necessarily valid scientific instruments. The Rorschach does have a specific scoring guide, which the TAT does not, but both are subjective instruments: The personality of the tester, especially if he or she is not specifically trained to do such testing, may influence the results. A student may have a "maladjusted" label attached to his school records, following him for years, because of misinterpretation of test results by an ill-trained tester or teacher. On the other hand, of course, a youngster who is indeed maladjusted may receive much-needed help as a result of the testing procedure.

Critics also raise objections on the grounds of violation of privacy. Some projective tests include questions about sexual practices or belief in God or relationships with parents; such questions, critics argue, are not relevant to school performance or ability to do a specific job. The argument is not resolved. A federal judge ruled in the spring of 1978 that psychological testing did not violate the rights of prospective firemen.

Child rearing

Freud's theories on the complexity of children's minds, on the role of unconscious drives, and on parent-child interaction have had a marked effect on American child-rearing practices. The effect became most pronounced in the 1940s and 1950s, in the aftermath of World War II and in the swing away from earlier regimentation in the nursery. (Behaviorist psychology, which emerged from the laboratory after Freud had developed his psychoanalytic theories, influenced the nursery first. Behaviorist theory and practice are described in Part III.)

Dr. Benjamin Spock, whose *Baby and Child Care* became

the bible for generations of American parents, was the leading but by no means the only psychoanalytically trained dispenser of advice in the postwar era. Then and now, Dr. Spock represented, above all, acceptance of children's emotional needs. He also reflected the view, expressed in 1950 at the Mid-Century White House Conference on Children and Youth, that parents can make mistakes as long as they love their children; feelings are more important than specific techniques.

Feelings, however, are interpreted within a Freudian framework. The child should know, for example, that angry feelings are perfectly normal. Angry feelings are acceptable, Dr. Spock advises in the 1957 edition of *Baby and Child Care*; angry actions are not. The child should be restrained from acting out aggression—but not made to feel guilty because he feels aggressive. Later interpretations of this advice—distortions, Dr. Spock would say—allowed, almost encouraged, children to act out all sorts of impulses, including dangerously destructive ones.

Spock said that it was all right to displace aggression, to hit a doll instead of your sister. Other people were not supposed to be hurt, but the aggression itself should be released. Otherwise, if instincts were thwarted, the child would not move on to the next stage of development. But the advice became garbled somewhere along the way. Some parents, afraid to thwart an instinct, never said "no." Children in these families sensed tacit permission to strike out at authority, both verbally and physically, in the interests of mental health. The permissive era has been attributed to Dr. Freud and to Dr. Spock, although Dr. Spock, at least, disclaims the responsibility. But even today, and perhaps not surprisingly, parents are confused by conflicting advice. Should it all "hang out"? Or should feelings be restrained in the interest of civilization? Dr. Spock, despite criticism of him in the 1960s, has always advocated a middle road.

Selma Fraiberg, a well-known psychoanalyst of children, has carried the Freudian message into American homes in even more direct terms. In her book *The Magic Years*, she speaks of the development of the ego in the preschool child. The ego, according to Freud, mediates between the biological drives of the id and the forces of reality which limit gratification. The ego, during childhood, gradually becomes strong enough to find a solution to the inevitable conflict. But that strength takes a while to develop, and parents, Fraiberg suggests, would do well to understand the course of development. A two-and-a-half-year-old, for instance, alone in the kitchen with a bowl of eggs, feels a strong desire to break the eggs. She reaches for them, but feels, quite rightly, that Mother (the externalized conscience in the young child) would disapprove. The solution, consistent with this stage of ego development: Mother returns to the kitchen to find the child, as Fraiberg puts it, "cheerfully plopping eggs on the linoleum and scolding herself sharply for each plop, 'NoNoNo. Mustn't dood it. NoNoNo. *Mustn't* dood it!' "

Sometimes, as children get a little older and more verbal, an imaginary playmate arrives on the scene. When guilt is transferred to the imaginary friend ("I didn't break the plate—*he* did"), the ego is beginning to achieve some control over the id. The dangerous impulses of the id are being recognized as subject, just barely, to control. Eventually, when the child's ego is strong enough, the id can be internalized and the imaginary friend disappears.

The Oedipus complex shows up in the writings of both Spock and Fraiberg. Spock speaks, in his early work and again in *Raising Children in a Difficult Time* (1974), of the romantic love boys have for their mothers and girls have for their fathers. This love, in the years between three and five, leads to intense rivalry with the parent of the same sex. It leads to jealousy of that parent. And it leads to guilt over the

37

intensity of the feeling. If something happens to the parent while the child has been wishing the parent's disappearance, the feelings of guilt may be intolerable. Even if nothing happens, as is usually the case, the child may be upset by the realization that he wants the parent out of the way. Spock's advice to parents: These feelings are normal; they should be neither encouraged nor punished; they will be outgrown.

Fraiberg gives essentially the same advice, pointing out that parental understanding can be a great help to the child in resolving such conflicts. The Oedipus complex is indeed a conflict for the child. Jimmy may want to dispose of his father so he can marry his mother—but he loves his father, at the same time, and is horrified at his own thoughts. The conflict is usually resolved by the time the child is five or six. Then, realizing, it seems, that he cannot take his father's place, he resolves to be like his father; the girl determines to be like her mother.

Meanwhile, while the conflict still rages, behavior resulting from Oedipal feelings can be very mystifying to parents. The little boy who feels guilty about wishing his father out of the way, for instance, may act up, unconsciously provoking his father to the point of punishment; once punished, the child can feel legitimately wronged, legitimately angry at his father. The child doesn't know why he acts this way. And the father, poor soul, can't figure out what brought on the rebellion. The psychoanalyst would recognize that misbehavior, guilt feelings, and bad dreams can, one and all, stem from an Oedipus conflict in the process of being repressed.

Parental love, according to Spock, overcomes parental ineptitude. Mothers and fathers can lose their tempers. A little boy can be punished for his misbehavior as long as the overall climate in the home is warm and supportive. At the same time, however, Freudians also say that single events can cause psychic harm. This concept—that children are fragile emotional beings easily damaged by traumatic events—places enormous responsibility on parental shoulders. So does the claim that individual personality is formed in the early interaction between parent and child.

That responsibility has been the subject of much recent criticism. One long-range study, for instance, clearly demonstrates that infants are born with recognizable differences in temperament. Nine characteristics, with extremes of behavior, were identified by Dr. Alexander Thomas and Dr. Stella Chess and their co-workers: motor activity, regularity or rhythmicity of behavior, distractibility, approach-withdrawal, adaptability, attention span and persistence, intensity of reaction, threshold of responsiveness, quality of mood. The adaptable infant, for instance, doesn't object to being bathed or changed; the nonadaptive infant resists. The active newborn moves often during sleep, wriggles when a diaper is being changed; the newborn who shows low activity level does not move very much at all. The baby with a long attention span and a high level of persistence repeatedly rejects water if he wants milk; the baby with a shorter attention span won't object too strenuously if offered a substitute.

What all this comes down to is that infants differ considerably. Some are placid, some volatile; some reject new experiences, others welcome them. These built-in temperamental differences, and the way that parents, with their own temperamental makeup, react to them, shape the child's emotional development. Early parent-child interaction is undeniably important, but the basic patterns of behavior are already established at birth. Parents are not totally responsible. "We have seen parents whose behavior should have created monsters," Dr. Chess wrote recently, "but produced marvels instead, and we have watched ideal parenting that produced horrors." Furthermore, much current research indicates that while basic temperament may be innate, the development of personality is not limited to childhood, or even

Temperamental Differences and Behavior in Childhood
(From *Scientific American*)

TEMPER-AMENTAL QUALITY	RATING	TWO MONTHS	TWO YEARS	TEN YEARS
Activity Level	High	Moves often in sleep. Wriggles when diaper is changed.	Climbs furniture. Explores. Gets in and out of bed while being put to sleep.	Plays ball and engages in other sports. Cannot sit still long enough to do homework.
	Low	Does not move when being dressed or during sleep.	Enjoys quiet play with puzzles. Can listen to records for hours.	Likes chess and reading. Eats very slowly.
Rhythmicity	Regular	Has been on four-hour feeding schedule since birth. Regular bowel movements.	Eats a big lunch each day. Always has a snack before bedtime.	Eats only at mealtimes. Sleeps the same amount of time each night.
	Irregular	Awakes at a different time each morning. Size of feedings varies.	Nap time changes from day to day. Toilet training is difficult because bowel movement is unpredictable.	Food intake varies. Falls asleep at a different time each night.
Distractibility	Distractible	Will stop crying for food if rocked. Stops fussing if given pacifier when diaper is being changed.	Will stop tantrum if another activity is suggested.	Needs absolute silence for homework. Has a hard time choosing a shirt in a store because they all appeal to him.
	Not Distractible	Will not stop crying when diaper is changed. Fusses after eating, even if rocked.	Screams if refused some desired object. Ignores mother's calling.	Can read a book while television set is at high volume. Does chores on schedule.
Approach/Withdrawal	Positive	Smiles and licks washcloth. Has always liked bottle.	Slept well the first time he stayed overnight at grandparents' house.	Went to camp happily. Loved to ski the first time.
	Negative	Rejected cereal the first time. Cries when strangers appear.	Avoids strange children in the playground. Whimpers first time at beach. Will not go into water.	Severely homesick at camp during first days. Does not like new activities.

Category	Rating			
Adaptability	Adaptive	Was passive during first bath; now enjoys bathing. Smiles at nurse.	Obeys quickly. Stayed contentedly with grandparents for a week.	Likes camp, although homesick during first days. Learns enthusiastically.
	Not Adaptive	Still startled by sudden, sharp noise. Resists diapering.	Cries and screams each time hair is cut. Disobeys persistently.	Does not adjust well to new school or new teacher; comes home late for dinner even when punished.
Attention Span and Persistence	Long	If soiled, continues to cry until changed. Repeatedly rejects water if he wants milk.	Works on a puzzle until it is completed. Watches when shown how to do something.	Reads for two hours before sleeping. Does homework carefully.
	Short	Cries when awakened but stops almost immediately. Objects only mildly if cereal precedes bottle.	Gives up easily if a toy is hard to use. Asks for help immediately if undressing becomes difficult.	Gets up frequently from homework for a snack. Never finishes a book.
Intensity of Reaction	Intense	Cries when diapers are wet. Rejects food vigorously when satisfied.	Yells if he feels excitement or delight. Cries loudly if a toy is taken away.	Tears up an entire page of homework if one mistake is made. Slams door of room when teased by younger brother.
	Mild	Does not cry when diapers are wet. Whimpers instead of crying when hungry.	When another child hit her, she looked surprised, did not hit back.	When a mistake is made in a model airplane, corrects it quietly. Does not comment when reprimanded.
Threshold of Responsiveness	Low	Stops sucking on bottle when approached.	Runs to door when father comes home. Must always be tucked tightly into bed.	Rejects fatty foods. Adjusts shower until water is at exactly the right temperature.
	High	Is not startled by loud noises. Takes bottle and breast equally well.	Can be left with anyone. Falls to sleep easily on either back or stomach.	Never complains when sick. Eats all foods.
Quality of Mood	Positive	Smacks lips when first tasting new food. Smiles at parents.	Plays with sister; laughs and giggles. Smiles when he succeeds in putting shoes on.	Enjoys new accomplishments. Laughs when reading a funny passage aloud.
	Negative	Fusses after nursing. Cries when carriage is rocked.	Cries and squirms when given haircut. Cries when mother leaves.	Cries when he cannot solve a homework problem. Very "weepy" if he does not get enough sleep.

to adolescence. Growth and change continue throughout life—and events in mid-life can affect the ego as strongly as events in childhood. Given this current insight, based on extended research, Freud's theories play a less significant role. They still play a part, but only a part, in today's understanding of human nature.

Freud and feminism

Freud has been criticized for his views on the development of personality in general. He has been criticized even more strongly in some quarters for his views on the development of personality in women.

It starts, as do all Freudian theories, in early childhood. Somewhere around the age of two-and-a-half or three, just as the Oedipus complex is moving into full gear, little boys and girls realize that they are not made alike. The girl thinks she is missing something and is in some way inferior; Freud called this penis envy. The boy thinks that the girl has been mutilated in an accident and that the same sort of accident could happen to him; Freud called this the castration complex. Both penis envy and the castration complex have long-range effects on the adult personality. Women, it is claimed, have a sense of inferiority and are always envious of men. Men, on the other hand, protective of their masculinity, are contemptuous of women. Women, in fact, also become contemptuous of women.

Both sexes may wind up with the unconscious feeling that, because they are not alike physically, they are not the same, not equal, in any respect. Psychoanalysts have until recently confirmed this view, insisting that men and women have different life roles to play. Those different roles allow little room for individual temperament. A "healthy" woman was defined as a happy wife and mother. Period. The desire for the male organ is supposed to change, with maturity, into the desire for a child. The woman who wants no child, or, worse yet, the woman who wants to combine a career with motherhood, is neurotic. That opinion lingers on. Some contemporary psychoanalysts, including Selma Fraiberg in her new book, *Every Child's Birthright*, speak of the fulfillment that both child and mother derive from full-time motherhood.

But women, just like men, are individuals. Some are competitive, some are independent, some are assertive. Some are fulfilled only if they work outside the home, others if they stay home full-time, others if they combine careers within the home and out. The most devastating legacy of Freudian theory, according to those who see the individuality of both male and female human beings, is its definition of normalcy. A "normal" adult and a "normal" male have long been defined by psychoanalysts as exactly the same thing; a "normal" female was something entirely different. It was normal for mature adults, i.e., men, to be interested in careers, to be independent, logical, and assertive. It was neurotic for a woman to display any of these same traits.

The inevitable result: Men who enjoyed their children were looked on with suspicion. Women with career ambitions were, until very recently, made to feel less than "real" women. If such a woman entered analysis, she was helped to overcome her "neurosis" and accept her role as a woman. Today, at least partly through the influence of the women's rights movement, many analysts have modified their views. They recognize that women, like men, can find fulfillment in work as well as in family. They see that men, like women, can be sensitive human beings. They see that people, both men and women, are three-dimensional rather than cardboard cutouts.

But even today Freud's legacy lingers on. Dr. Spock wrote, as recently as 1974:

"Freud taught—and I still believe—that girls acquire in early childhood an unconscious sense of bodily inferiority, to one degree or another, from a misunderstanding of the physical sexual differences. Of course, feminists consider that Freud was so biased against women as to be almost totally unreliable. I admit he has the usual male prejudices, but I don't think that this discredits his basic, verifiable discoveries."

Dr. Spock goes on to discuss the lifelong conditioning that so often makes women feel inferior. This lifelong social influence—the attitudes of parents and teachers, portrayals in books and on television—are indeed the crux of the matter. But Freud's theories legitimized this treatment of women for many years, to the detriment of both men and women.

Sigmund Freud and the theories he put forth have had enormous influence on our civilization. But it must be remembered that Freud was a product of his time, a time in which masculinity was the cultural and sexual norm. The repressed sexuality that was the cornerstone of his theory was perhaps typical of upper-middle-class Victorian Europe. So was the subordinate position of women. Neither is necessarily appropriate to a late-twentieth-century view of human nature.

PART III

Behaviorism: Psychology in the Laboratory

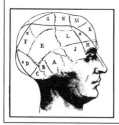

B. F. Skinner:
A theory of learning

If your small brother has an unreasoning fear of large furry dogs, do you think it's because he has a deep-seated and unresolved Oedipal conflict? Or do you think it's probably because he once had a frightening experience with just such an animal? Psychoanalysts of the Freudian school look for underlying neurotic conflict to explain behavior; behaviorist psychologists look at the behavior itself. The difference is crucial in twentieth-century psychology.

Behaviorism, unlike psychoanalysis, is concerned only with observable behavior. Behaviorist psychologists believe, in fact, that personality consists of learned behavior. There is no room in this theory for unconscious drives; there is no room for conscious intent. Personality is simply behavior controlled, or conditioned, by environmental forces. There are two forms of conditioning: classical and operant.

45

In classical conditioning, technically called respondent conditioning, an animal (human or not) automatically responds to some stimulus. A famous example is Pavlov's dog: The animal, which had salivated when presented with food (an involuntary reflex; we all do it), began to salivate in anticipation of food when it heard Pavlov's footsteps. When Pavlov became aware of this development, in his research into digestive processes, he redirected his research into the process of conditioning. By ringing a bell each time food was presented to the dog, he quickly conditioned the animal to salivate at the sound of a bell, whether or not food was present. A similar experience might happen to you: If you are accustomed to having lunch when the school bell signals a particular period, you may feel distinctly hungry at, or just before, the sound of that bell; you may even hear your stomach growl.

Operant conditioning is a little more complicated; it deals with voluntary action rather than involuntary reflex. Its basis: Behavior which has positive consequences, which is reinforced in some way, is likely to recur. If pizza tastes good, in a simple example, you will probably order pizza again. If a classmate tells you you look particularly well in a certain shirt, you may very well wear that shirt more often than others. If your parents bestow lavish praise when your room is neat, you may—just may—keep it that way. Every aspect of your behavior, from what you wear to how you study to your relationship with family and friends, is based, in the behaviorist view, on operant conditioning. Every aspect of human behavior, from making love to making war, is, in the behaviorist view, a product of operant conditioning.

There are many psychologists in the behaviorist camp today. The most important is probably B. F. Skinner of Harvard. But before Skinner, another behaviorist had considerable impact. His name: John B. Watson.

Watson: "Children are made, not born"

John Locke, a seventeenth-century English philosopher, believed that the human mind, at birth, is nothing more than a tabula rasa, a blank slate waiting to be inscribed by the world. John Watson brought this view into the scientific laboratory and into the twentieth century. One of the first to view psychology as an objective science whose goal, as he put it in 1913, "is the prediction and control of behavior," Watson was the founder of American behaviorist psychology. He coined the word *behaviorism,* in fact, to reflect his belief that the only valid data for psychological research are observable behaviors—not mind or drives or the unconscious.

Watson believed that infants are born with a minimum repertoire of basic reflexes, ready to be molded into a human being much as a lump of clay is ready to be molded by the potter's wheel. Everything beyond the basic reflexes, every possible form of behavior from the simple to the complex, is brought about by conditioning. Walking, for example, is described by psychologist Adelaide Bry as "an interconnected series of conditioned reflex movements in which each movement serves as the conditioned stimulus for the movement that follows it." Weight placed on one foot is a stimulus for weight being placed on the other foot. That's walking in terms of classical conditioning. In operant terms, walking takes place because it is reinforced—it has positive consequences. The infant learns to walk, keeps at it despite numerous falls along the way, because the act of walking gives him some control over his surroundings. The older child may walk because the destination, such as a friend's house, provides the reinforcement. A desk-bound executive may walk to and from her job for the exercise. Either the destination or the act of walking itself can provide reinforcement.

Even the basic reflexes, including what we might call complex emotions unique to human beings, can be described (according to Watson) only in terms of observable

47

behavior. Feelings are subject to misinterpretation; behavior alone can be objectively described. You can say that your little brother is crying; you cannot say what he feels. Similarly, love is said to exist when one human being exhibits "approach behavior" toward another. Love, in this view, is conditioned by one person's behavior toward another. It is made up initially of a pattern of responses reinforced in the infant by a parent's touch and voice.

Because all newborn human beings, in this view, start with the same basic endowment (Watson discounted inherited qualities), he could say in 1928, in what has become a famous statement: "Give me a dozen healthy infants, well-formed, and my own special world to bring them up in and I'll guarantee to take any one at random and train him to become any type of specialist I might select—into a doctor, lawyer, artist, merchant-chief, and yes, even into beggarman and thief, regardless of his talents, penchants, tendencies, abilities, vocations and race of ancestors."

That was quite a promise. Watson never did have the opportunity to make good on it, perhaps because mothers were reluctant to give him their children. But he did make history with one case, the famous case of "little Albert." Albert, a healthy child with a placid temperament, was under a year old when Watson ran him through a series of tests which indicated that he had no fears whatsoever. Watson took care of that. He embarked on a program of classical conditioning. Every time Albert reached toward a white rat, a nice furry object, a steel bar out of sight behind the child's head was struck with a hammer. Naturally enough, the child flinched and cried. It didn't take long, just about eight trials, before the child flinched and cried at the rat alone, withdrawing in apparent terror at the sight of the animal. Albert learned his lesson well: He became terrified of rabbits, cotton wool, fur coats, and the beard on a mask of Santa Claus.

Watson intended to condition Albert to rid him of his

acquired fears, but Albert's mother had apparently had enough. The child was removed from the laboratory, leaving Watson to speculate that Freudians would have a field day, in later years, tracing the source of his fears to a repressed sexual conflict.

Conditioning to rid a child of specific fears could be done, however, as Mary Cover Jones later demonstrated. She worked with a young child named Peter who, coincidentally, was afraid of both rats and rabbits. By gradually bringing a caged rabbit into a room where Peter was happily playing with other children, then, over a period of days, bringing the rabbit closer and closer, Jones eliminated the fear. In behaviorist terms, the stimulus which had caused the fear (the rabbit) was associated with a reinforcer in the form of a pleasant situation (the company of other children), so that a new conditioned response took effect.

Watson eventually left psychology and turned to advertising. If you find yourself responding favorably to a particular brand of shampoo, it may well be because of the behaviorist theories Watson applied to this field. His experimental work, however, made a long-lasting mark on psychology, both inside and outside the laboratory. It reached into many homes, and influenced the way in which many of your grandparents brought up your parents; the next chapter has the details. And it influenced the continuing research of many psychologists, among them B. F. Skinner.

Skinner: "Happiness . . . is a by-product of operant reinforcement"

"Freudian dynamisms or defense mechanisms . . . are not psychic processes taking place in the depths of the mind, conscious or unconscious; they are the effects of contingencies of reinforcement, almost always involving punishment."

What does this mean? Is the jargon of behaviorism any

more meaningful than the jargon of psychoanalysis? Skinner, who has been working at Harvard since 1948, thinks it is. He has gone well beyond Watson in applying behaviorist theories to human actions; in the process he has left Freudian theory far behind.

Skinner started working with animals, specifically with three baby squirrels. When peanuts were hung from a tree branch by a string, he found, the squirrels would pull on the string to reach the peanuts. From these early experiments in Harvard Yard, Skinner moved into the laboratory, concentrating his research efforts on operant conditioning and working primarily with rats and pigeons. He worked with these animals in an experimental cage which has come to be called, appropriately enough, a Skinner box. The essential ingredients of the Skinner box are a food tray, a food-releasing mechanism, and, most important, some manipulative device. The box may also contain a light and/or a grid floor which can conduct a mild electric charge. But the essential ingredient is the manipulative device, a bar or key which the animal manipulates with paw or beak in order to release the food.

Skinner boxes are now used in experimental laboratories all over the world as both observation rooms and teaching chambers. They allow scientists to see what animals will do in certain situations. When a rat has accidentally pressed the bar which releases a food pellet, for example, how soon will it do so again? And they allow scientists to train the animals, by deliberately providing reinforcement when the animal performs a desired action, thereby increasing the likelihood that the animal will perform it again.

Behavioral theory (and practice) is based on the fundamental idea that all behaviors are maintained by their consequences. Behavior which is reinforced by its consequences tends to be repeated. When the rat in the Skinner box receives food for pressing the bar, he is likely to press the bar again; when you are praised for keeping your room neat, you are more likely to do so in the future. Behavior which is not reinforced is not as likely to be repeated. If pressing the bar does not bring reinforcement in the form of food, the rat's movements will be random; if no one notices or remarks on your attempts at neatness, you will probably assume the effort was wasted.

What is reinforcement? That all depends. For laboratory animals, the primary positive reinforcement is food or water. Providing a nugget of food each and every time a rat successfully runs a maze will increase the likelihood that the rat will run the maze. For domestic animals, social reinforcement also counts. Your dog may be conditioned by food if you offer a dog biscuit each time it obeys a command, but it will also respond to a pat on the head and your approving voice. For human beings, both primary and social reinforcers can be effective. A piece of candy after dinner may reinforce good table manners in a three-year-old—and a gold star may reinforce the toothbrushing behavior which will counteract the candy. Good grades may reinforce your study habits. Praise may reinforce neatness.

If it is to be effective, the particular reinforcer, whatever it is, has to mean something to the subject. If you don't like movies, the promise of a movie will not reinforce your behavior. But nothing is a reinforcer, in strict behaviorist terms, because it "means something." It is a reinforcer only because it increases the likelihood that the behavior will be repeated. Behaviorists deal only with what can be observed.

If it is to be effective, too, whatever it is, the reinforcer must be applied immediately. If the rat in the Skinner box presses the bar, then runs to the other side of the cage, then receives the nugget of food, the behavior that is being reinforced is not pressing the bar but running to the other side of the cage. If your dog sits on command and then, before you reward it, begins to bark, the reward will reinforce the act of barking. If a history paper is graded and returned in short order, the grade may spur you on to further effort; if there is a long delay, the reinforcement value of the grade may be lost.

When a new behavior is being taught, reinforcement should be continuous. Every single time the subject performs the desired behavior, reinforcement should be provided. Every single time the rat presses the bar, food should be provided. Once the new behavior is well established, however, reinforcement can be intermittent or occasional: The pellet of food may be provided after every five or six bar pressings instead of after every single one. Intermittent reinforcement may be on a time or number or random basis. Examples: Pay per hour on your part-time job is time-based reinforcement. A prize for each five magazine subscriptions sold is number-based reinforcement. A win at the one-armed bandit in Las Vegas, unpredictable in any sense, is random reinforcement.

Intermittent reinforcement, whatever the schedule, reinforces behavior. Otherwise, if reinforcement is removed altogether from a previously conditioned response, the result is extinction, the "unlearning" of the behavior. The gambler who never wins will be far less likely to continue gambling; one win may be all he needs to keep on going. Conditioned behavior, unless maintained by intermittent reinforcement, is temporary. In fact, Pavlov called it condition*al* behavior. The name has changed, but the principle remains the same.

Reinforcement may also be negative. In behaviorist terms, negative reinforcement is operative upon its removal—the less it takes place, the more likely the response is to occur. This is not the same as punishment, which acts to decrease rather than increase the target behavior. Negative reinforcers, also sometimes called aversive stimuli, are primarily laboratory techniques: Researchers can induce an animal to enter a particular part of its cage either by offering it food (a positive reinforcement) or by removing an electric charge (a negative reinforcement).

Skinner has accomplished some remarkable feats with his rats and pigeons. He has taught pigeons to play Ping-Pong and, on the more serious side, to pilot missiles. During World War II, pigeons were conditioned in the laboratory to peck steadily at the image of a target on a screen. If they did so in the nose of a moving missile, the researchers believed, they would keep the missile on course. The pigeons were never actually put to work, but the training was successful.

Such sophisticated tasks are taught through the process of shaping. While you can wait for a rat to accidentally press a bar, and then provide reinforcement, the rat will be more likely to press the bar in the first place if any movement in that direction is reinforced. At first the rat might receive a food pellet when it moves toward the side of the cage where the bar is located. Then the rat might have to come within six inches of the bar to receive its reward. The next step might involve standing next to the bar. The final step in this slow and intricate dance would be actually pressing the bar.

You can't wait until a pigeon independently guides a missile to its target. You must shape such complex behavior gradually, one step at a time, by providing reinforcement whenever a movement, no matter how slight, is made in the desired direction. The first time the pigeon even moves its head to the right, for instance, it receives a reward.

Skinner describes how the principles of shaping were discovered. In a light moment during the serious research of World War II, he and his colleagues decided to teach a pigeon to bowl, to send a wooden ball down a miniature alley toward a set of miniature pins. The researchers decided to provide a food pellet as soon as the pigeon took a swipe at the ball with its beak. After a lengthy wait, however, the research team became impatient. They then decided to reinforce any response which appeared to be even the smallest step in the right direction. As soon as they did so, initially rewarding the pigeon for simply looking at the wooden ball, they were amazed by the results. "In a few minutes," Skinner reported, "the ball was caroming off the walls of the box as if the pigeon had been a champion squash player."

Reinforcement, and the step-by-step shaping of behavior, is not limited to the laboratory. Human behavior is also shaped by its consequences. Skinner, in fact, defines Freud's elements of the unconscious—the id, the superego, and the ego—in behaviorist terms. The id, he says, is "man's 'unregenerate nature,' derived from his innate suscepti-bilities to reinforcement, most of them almost necessarily in conflict with the interests of others." The superego is the Judeo-Christian conscience, the internalized interests of other people. And the ego, in this behaviorist framework, acts in accordance with the practical contingencies of daily life.

These practical contingencies in day-to-day life are often accidental. Praise is a powerful social reinforcer—but parents are not necessarily consistent in praising the good behavior of small children. Sometimes they fail to notice. Sometimes reinforcement is misapplied. The teacher who scolds a rowdy youngster while ignoring a studious one (as-suming perhaps that the studious one needs no attention) may actually be reinforcing rowdy behavior. Sometimes su-perstition arises out of accidental reinforcement: If you wore a particular hat to the game the day your team finally won, you may wear that hat to the next game. If the team wins again, a superstition—built on a reinforcer—may be launched.

When reinforcement is deliberate rather than accidental, it becomes what psychologists call behavior modification. The underlying premise is simple: If behavior is conditioned by environmental forces, as behavioral psychologists believe, then those forces can be deliberately manipulated to create desirable behavior patterns and eliminate undesirable patterns. Behavior modification may be applied by others: Your teachers may try to deal with discipline problems in the classroom by modifying the behavior of students. And it may be applied, as the next chapter will show, by the individual concerned.

The behavior modifier does not rely on accidental or random consequences. He sets out deliberately and systematically to provide the consequences which will shape behavior. First the specific behavior which is to be modified is selected, then a reinforcer which is likely to work with the particular individual is chosen (often with the agreement of the subject), and then a schedule of reinforcement is implemented.

An important element of any behavior modification program is selective attention: The modifier must ignore undesirable behavior, as difficult as it may be to do so, and concentrate attention on the desired behavior. This is almost contrary to human nature. The mother who is chatting with a friend over a cup of tea is not likely to pay much attention to the toddler playing quietly nearby. She is likely to pay attention, especially if she is embarrassed in front of her friend, if her child suddenly bites his playmate. A teacher, similarly, is more likely to pay attention to the disruptive student than to the studious one.

The behavior modifier, however, would reinforce desirable behavior by, at the very least, praising the toddler who is playing quietly or the student who is attending to work. Such selective attention can forestall problem behavior. Once problem behavior is established, the parent or teacher faces a more difficult task. Then the modifier must embark on a deliberate program, systematically reinforcing behavior which approximates the desired behavior until new behavior patterns are shaped and established. If, for example, a teacher is annoyed by a student who keeps hopping out of his seat, the teacher should reinforce this student for in-seat behavior; the reinforcement should be very frequent at first, perhaps after three minutes in the seat, and gradually decrease in frequency.

The reinforcement itself may consist of praise or attention, or it may be something tangible. A token system is sometimes used in classrooms, where pieces of cardboard with assigned points may be accumulated and turned in for specific privileges. A token system may also be used at home, where gold stars may be awarded to a three-year-old each time teeth are brushed. A program of self-modification might include a favorite TV program after a day with no cigarettes. But, as in the laboratory, the schedule of reinforcement must be consistently followed.

The principles of behaviorism do work. They work particularly well when subjects have volunteered, but they work even when people are unaware that they are the subjects of an experiment. Guy Lefrancois, an educational psychologist, tells a story of his own student days. After learning the principles of behaviorism, he and some fellow students decided to shape the behavior of their teacher. They nodded approvingly at his lectures whenever he paced the floor while talking; within four lectures, he paced at a steady rate. Then they decided to nod approvingly only when he spoke from a particular corner of the room; he obediently followed suit— all the while unaware that his behavior was being shaped in accordance with the principles he had taught.

Reinforcement is very powerful. But it can have a two-way effect. There's a cartoon that has one rat, in a Skinner box, saying to another: "Boy, have I got this guy trained! Every time I press the lever, he gives me some food." If every time you clean up your room your mother becomes particularly generous, who is training whom?

When a group of California high-school students learned

behavior modification techniques, they used them to reinforce positive behavior on the part of teachers, smiling at and praising teachers who were helpful and fair. They particularly enjoyed telling teachers that they finally understood a specific subject area, understood it because it had been so well explained by the individual teacher. In this case, reported by *Psychology Today* magazine a couple of years ago, the students were convinced that they had engineered a change in teacher behavior. Their teachers, on the other hand, were also pleased with the results—but believed that the project had changed the behavior of the students.

Such situations are amusing. But there are some serious questions about behaviorist psychology and behavior modification, questions about human nature and about the issue of control.

In terms of human nature, some observers are disturbed by the behaviorists' seeming negation of the human mind, of intelligence and spirituality, and, above all else, of freedom. Freedom and free will, according to Skinner, are nothing but illusions; like it or not, we are controlled by the conditions of our environment. Since this is so, it is up to us to arrange those conditions so that the maximum amount of good results, so that people will not be reinforced for polluting the atmosphere or for making war. Through behavioral technology based on operant conditioning, Skinner is convinced, we can create a peaceful, productive world. All we have to do is arrange the appropriate reinforcement for socially useful behavior.

If you grant this power of behavioral technology (and many people wonder whether the entire human population is as trainable as a flock of pigeons), you are probably still troubled by another issue: Who controls the contingencies of reinforcement? Who decides what behavior is desirable? Who decides who shall decide? Who, in short, shall have the ultimate power to control human behavior?

Aldous Huxley had one answer. In *Brave New World* the government, a monolithic dictatorial central government of the world, makes all the decisions. It decides before any human being is born what that human's destiny will be. It conditions that human being, both before birth, in the Bottling Rooms which replaced human parents, and after birth, in the nursery to which each level of human being was assigned. Those to be sent as adults to hot climates were born with a horror of the cold; those designed as menial laborers were conditioned in the nursery to dislike flowers and books. There is no free will in *Brave New World*. And that, Huxley writes, is the secret of happiness: "liking what you've *got* to do. All conditioning aims at that: making people like their unescapable social destiny."

Control over behavior in our society has not reached this level. But behavior is nonetheless controlled to some extent. It is controlled haphazardly, if not deliberately, in the classroom and in the mental hospital; in the prison and in the home. And it is controlled inconsistently. One teacher may reinforce docile and obedient behavior; another approves active participation and seeking after information. What happens to the students as they move from one of these teachers to the other? Which teacher is right? Should a school principal have the power to decide which methods to follow? Or should a teacher tolerate (or try to tolerate) assorted behaviors in the classroom, behaviors reflecting the individual characteristics of individual children rather than the teacher's preference?

Critics of behaviorism contend that behaviorism is both simplistic and manipulative, a denial of human dignity in the interests of efficiency and conformity. But B. F. Skinner believes that the principles of behaviorism can and should be put to work to make the world a better place. One way or the other, good or bad, behaviorism has had a profound influence on twentieth-century psychology.

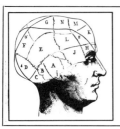

Putting behaviorism
to work

Two hundred years ago Benjamin Franklin, determined to improve his character, embarked on a program of self-modification. He didn't call it that, of course. But, as described in a recent article in *Psychology Today*, that's exactly what Franklin did. He compiled a list of thirteen "virtues," including such qualities as sincerity and justice and humility, and kept track each day of the number of times he missed his self-set goal.

Franklin was not completely successful—he recognized, in ironic fact, that if he did manage to achieve humility, he would probably be proud of his success—but behavioral principles, whether self-applied or applied by others, are powerful implements. They have become even greater implements as twentieth-century behaviorism has moved from the laboratory into our homes and our schools and our lives.

Benjamin Franklin's Behavior Modification Diary

TEMPERANCE.

Eat not to dulness: drink not to elevation.

	Sun.	M.	T.	W.	Th.	F.	S.
Tem.							
Sil.	•	•		•		•	
Ord.	•	•	•		•	•	•
Res.		•				•	
Fru.		•				•	
Ind.			•				
Sinc.							
Jus.							
Mod.							
Clea.							
Tran.							
Chas.							
Hum.							

TEMPERANCE
Eat not to dulness. Drink not to elevation.

SILENCE
Speak not but what may benefit others or yourself. Avoid trifling conversation.

ORDER
Let all your things have their places. Let each part of your business have its time.

RESOLUTION
Resolve to perform what you ought. Perform without fail what you resolve.

FRUGALITY
Make no expense but to do good to others or yourself; i.e., waste nothing.

INDUSTRY
Lose no time. Be always employed in something useful. Cut off all unnecessary actions.

SINCERITY
Use no hurtful deceit. Think innocently and justly; and, if you speak, speak accordingly.

JUSTICE
Wrong none by doing injuries or omitting the benefits that are your duty.

MODERATION
Avoid extremes. Forbear resenting injuries so much as you think they deserve.

CLEANLINESS
Tolerate no uncleanness in body, clothes or habitation.

TRANQUILITY
Be not disturbed at trifles or at accidents common or unavoidable.

CHASTITY
Rarely use venery but for health or offspring—never to dulness, weakness, or the injury of your own or another's peace or reputation.

HUMILITY
Imitate Jesus and Socrates.

Behaviorism at home

Operant conditioning—the rule that behavior is influenced by its consequences—has always been part of child rearing. "Train up a child in the way he should go . . ." is only one expression of the eternal belief that what parents do makes a difference. But the systematic application of behavioral principles, the tidal wave that inundated the American nursery in the 1930s, was something new. That tidal wave was generated to a large extent by John B. Watson.

In 1928, some years after little Albert was conditioned to fear animals (and some time after Watson left the laboratory to join the world of advertising), Watson published a book. *Psychological Care of Infant and Child* gave a glow of scientific respectability to the idea that children could be conditioned, could be trained to behave in socially acceptable ways. American parents seemed ready to accept the message, and your parents (like this author) may well have been brought up, at least in part, according to behaviorist principles.

Why the enthusiasm? Well, in addition to making child-rearing seem as manageable as animal training, Watson's behaviorism carried an implicit all-American message that every child could grow up to be President. If heredity doesn't count, if inner drives and motivation don't exist, and if all that does count is the process of conditioning, then all men (and all women) are indeed created equal, with equal opportunity for a glorious future. As B. F. Skinner put it much more recently, there is nothing "bad" about people who behave badly. It's a defective social environment that is at fault—and defective social environments can be changed.

Such optimism, however, like all strong medicine, sometimes has unlooked-for side effects. If behaviorism gives parents great power, it gives them equally great responsibility. If parents can shape children to a desired image, if parents are responsible for the social environment in which the child grows, then parents are to blame if the children are not "perfect." This aspect of behaviorism—the guilt it instilled in many parents—may not have been immediately noticeable in the first flush of excitement about its possibilities.

Watson's theories, in any event, made their mark on the nursery in several ways: early toilet training; strict feeding schedules; and a bare minimum of love and attention. Few American parents followed Watson's advice to the letter. But most were influenced, at least to some extent, by his beliefs. In some areas the influence continues.

Toilet training, for instance, is viewed not as a situation fraught with peril for the formation of character, but as a matter of simple conditioning: If the child and the toilet are brought together at regular and frequent intervals, with appropriate reinforcement when the child performs—a hug, for instance, and ample praise, as in "What a big boy!"—training should be accomplished by six to eight months of age. Today most doctors recognize that babies at this age do not yet have the necessary muscle control. If a baby happens to have regular movements, and if the mother happens to catch them, she may think the baby is trained; actually, it is the mother who is trained to do the catching. Most children are not able to control their bodily functions until they are past two years of age. Yet even in the 1970s a child-psychology text suggests that parents pay close attention to pre-elimination signals, pick the child up as rapidly as possible, and try to have the process finished in the bathroom. The parent should entice the child to sit there "with all sorts of attractions and rewards," and reward the child who does the expected.

In the 1920s and 1930s many middle-class babies were placed on a four-hour feeding schedule right after birth. The four hours was an arbitrary selection, adopted because it seemed to be the natural rhythm of many babies. But it wasn't the natural rhythm of *all* babies; as we realize today,

63

there is great individual variation. Yet many a mother, afraid to go against the advice of the "experts," listened in misery as a two- or three-week-old infant cried in hunger. Parents were not supposed to feed their children except on schedule; they were also not supposed to pick infants up between feedings. The same regularity, later on, was supposed to apply to family meals: Six o'clock supper should mean 6:00 supper, not 5:50 or 6:05 or, worse yet, 6:15.

Mothers who were more sure of themselves—or grandmothers who had never heard such nonsense—fed or cuddled babies when they cried. Some had good reason. As anthropologist Margaret Mead has explained, her mother agreed that one shouldn't pick up a crying child. But, Mead's mother went on, her babies were good babies who would cry only if something was wrong. And if something is wrong, a child should be picked up and comforted.

But it wasn't easy to go against the prevailing wisdom. And the prevailing wisdom, Watson's wisdom, held that babies could be easily "spoiled." We hear echoes of this today: "Don't pick up the baby when he cries. Let him cry it out. You don't want to spoil him." But today's echoes pale beside Watson's dictates. Watson really would have preferred to take children away from their parents, to be raised in scientifically pure surroundings uncontaminated by love. Lacking popular support for this position, he settled for telling parents that they should never, under any circumstances, cuddle their children. Instead, he sternly advised: "Treat them as though they were young adults. . . . Let your behavior always be objective and kindly firm. Never hug and kiss them, never let them sit in your lap. If you must, kiss them once on the forehead when they say good night. Shake hands with them in the morning. . . ."

It's interesting to compare this advice to contemporary awareness of children's emotional needs. Where Watson advised calm detachment, most psychologists in the 1970s are emphasizing the infant's need for bonding, for a close physical and emotional relationship with parents, starting as soon as possible after the moment of birth. Current thinking stems in part from Freud's realization that children do have innate feelings and emotions; they are not simply lumps of clay to be molded as the potter desires.

Yet behaviorism lingers on. After temporary displacement by Freudian theories in the 1940s and 1950s (Freud lived earlier, but his ideas didn't reach into American nurseries until mid-century), behaviorism, with its emphasis on fast and practical solutions, is again in vogue. Freud's theories are still heard, however, and advice is sometimes contradictory. "Let your baby suck his thumb," the Freudian psychologist might say; "this will satisfy the innate urge to suck, and forestall thumb sucking or other forms of oral gratification in later life." "*Don't* let your infant suck his thumb," the behaviorist is more likely to say; "if you prevent the sucking habit from being learned, less thumb sucking will take place." When you see an infant happily sucking away, that infant's parents, consciously or not, have been influenced by the Freudian view. When you see an infant wearing mittens in the middle of summer, you can be reasonably sure that his parents, whether they know it or not, are implementing behaviorist principles in an effort to prevent thumb sucking.

Once a habit is formed, it's another story. Then behaviorists recommend operant conditioning to substitute desirable behavior for the undesirable habit. Thumb sucking, while not necessarily a "bad habit" in an infant, becomes increasingly undesirable to many parents as a child grows older. Instead of resorting to mittens or evil-tasting substances or adhesive tape on the offending thumb, behaviorists would suggest a threefold procedure: Pinpoint the behavior you want to alter; record how frequently the behavior occurs; pick a consequence for the behavior, one that can be applied immediately and consistently.

If the target behavior is thumb sucking, the parent should look at the circumstances in which it occurs. If, for instance, it seems to occur solely when the child is overtired, a nap might do the trick. If it occurs when the child is bored, some pleasant diversion would be in order. In any case, the parent should offer the child a specific positive reinforcer whenever the child refrains from sucking the thumb for a specified period of time. The reinforcer might be a coloring book, if the child likes coloring books, or it might be a token toward something special—an afternoon at a ball game or the circus or whatever. Whatever it is, reinforcement should be supplied immediately.

The same principle applies to punishment. If a parent arrives home to find that a lamp was smashed earlier in the day, behaviorists say, it would be a mistake to confront the child with the evidence and then punish him. The right move, harder for parents to implement, requires being with the child, anticipating misbehavior—such as seeing when the child is about to throw a ball in the living room—and redirecting the behavior on the spot. Delayed punishment does no good. Reinforcement, whether it is intended to increase a desired behavior or remove an offending behavior, is effective only if it takes place as the behavior occurs.

But behaviorism can also be used, and often is, as a motivational device. With gold stars on a chart to indicate completion of piano practice, with monetary rewards for good grades in school, with a promised television program for display of proper table manners—with planned positive consequences for behavior of all kinds, in short—some parents are implementing behavioral principles. In doing so, they hope that the behavior will eventually become its own reward, so that reinforcement will become unnecessary. If reinforcement is to become unnecessary in the long run, however, it must be carefully planned: constant at first, then intermittent, then not at all.

66

Behaviorism in the schools

Any situation in which a group of individuals is controlled by others is fertile ground for behavioral techniques. Most highly structured programs of behavior modification are to be found in the tightly controlled classrooms and institutions established to meet the special needs of the mentally retarded. Institutionalized children, for instance, have been successfully toilet trained, while institutionalized adults have been conditioned to come to meals on time. But you may find examples of behaviorism in your own classroom as well.

Many elements of behaviorism, labeled as such or not, have always been found in the classroom. Positive reinforcement, for example, takes place all the time, in the form of praise for a well-thought-out question, gold stars (again!) for a neat notebook, free time when an assignment is completed, good grades for good work, and so on. When such reinforcement is accidental, it is usually inconsistent: Whether or not a teacher appreciates your question and praises you for it may depend on what other students are doing, the weather, and the mood of the teacher. When such reinforcement is accidental, it is often misapplied as well: The teacher who sits a wrongdoer in the corner is calling attention to the wrongdoer and thereby reinforcing his behavior.

Consistent and purposeful application of behavioral principles is more likely to be found in the ordinary classroom when that classroom is the scene of discipline problems. In one such chaotic classroom, where a series of substitute teachers had resulted in third-graders constantly out of their seats, sharpening pencils, wandering around, and talking, a behavior modification consultant brought order to the scene. She observed the situation, then devised a simple plan. A bell was rung, unannounced, two or three times in each class period. Any child who happened to be seated when the bell rang received a token, which could later be exchanged for candy. Within a week, out-of-seat incidents had dropped from seventeen per hour to two per hour.

The teacher who deliberately uses behavioral principles must be consistent; your praiseworthy answer should always receive praise. This teacher will also add some techniques to the repertoire of hit-or-miss reinforcement. In addition to consistent reinforcement of completed work and orderly behavior, he will reinforce steps along the way and thereby shape the desired response: Your first gold star may be awarded for a notebook page just slightly less sloppy than usual, the next for a relatively neat page, and so on, until neatness becomes self-reinforcing and gold stars are no longer necessary. In addition to praising good work and good behavior, the teacher will ignore misbehavior: The rowdy student will not be made to sit in the front of the room, where he can make faces at his classmates. In addition to free time when work is completed, the teacher may impose "time out" for not working or for rowdy behavior; this is time in isolation, where there is nothing to do but work.

There are also two specific instructional programs based on behavioral principles: contracts and programmed instruction. When a contract is used, teacher and student together work out an agreement designed to bring about desired behavior. Together they identify the behavior which is to change and select reinforcers which will be effective. A first-grader may sign a contract in which he agrees to stay in his seat during the reading lesson in exchange for fifteen minutes in which to listen to records later in the day. A high-school student may agree to get homework in on time in exchange for the privilege of working with a group on a particular assignment. As always, the reinforcer is delivered after the desired response, in exchange for actual behavior and not the promise of a behavior.

Programmed instruction began when B. F. Skinner visited his daughter's elementary-school arithmetic class in the early

1950s. Skinner, appalled by what he saw as mind-destroying waste in conventional methods of instruction, decided that children could learn arithmetic (and other subjects as well) the way pigeons learn Ping-Pong, through step-by-step conditioning. He thereupon devised the first teaching machine, designed to shape behavior through reinforcement; the reinforcement, instead of a food pellet or grain of corn, is the right answer. Information is presented in very small units; when each unit is mastered, the student moves on to the next. Mastery is demonstrated through providing the right answers to the questions which appear at each step of the way. If mastery is not demonstrated, the student backtracks until the material is learned. Students don't have to wait until a test paper has been marked and returned, sometimes after a week or two or three; reinforcement is immediate. And students don't move ahead until material is firmly grasped, thus eliminating the otherwise all-too-likely possibility of erecting a shaky superstructure on insecure foundations.

Programmed instruction can take a variety of forms. It can be presented in Skinner's original form, the teaching machine. This is a simple box, with a window panel, which contains the program on a roll of paper; the user turns a knob to reveal each succeeding question and answer. It can be woven into the text of a book, so that questions, followed by the correct answers, appear after each small unit of information. The student is supposed to mask the answer until he has supplied his own; in some books the student is tracked from page to page, so that answers are not immediately apparent. And programmed instruction can be implemented through printed or mimeographed worksheets. Individually Prescribed Instruction (IPI), which you may have encountered, is a highly structured form of individual instruction based on the principles of behaviorism. IPI subject matter, such as mathematics, is broken into a series of small sequential steps; the student moves to the next step, the next worksheet, only after competence is demonstrated. The demonstration of competence, through constant testing, tells the teacher how the student is doing, and at the same time provides reinforcement for the student.

Programmed instruction appeared for a while to be an answer to all kinds of educational problems. It looked so perfect, in fact, that some teachers worried about losing their jobs to machines. But programming, although it is useful for individualizing some areas of instruction, is not going to take over education. It has been found useful in conveying small units of factual information, in mathematics and spelling, but less useful in transmitting creative ideas, in history and literature. And even in the area of factual information, it can be very tedious to produce and to study any particular program. If units of instruction are too large, the trial-and-error process of selecting the right answers will take too long. If units are too small, the learner can easily become bored.

Behaviorism in our lives

Although the glitter of behaviorism has faded in some respects, it still holds great promise. Behaviorist principles, with their focus on solutions through action, are being applied in a great many ways. Businessmen, for instance, have discovered the power of positive reinforcement: If you praise a shipping clerk for packaging your product so that it survives shipping without breakage, packages are more likely to be correctly wrapped. If you base pay directly on job performance, performance generally improves.

A relatively new application is with animals, not with pigeons in the laboratory but with pet dogs who have picked up habits which disrupt the family. An animal psychologist may work directly with the pet, or with the pet owner. In one instance, two dogs, previously congenial occupants of the same household, began to fight. It got to the point where the fighting was incessant. Punishment did no good. The psychologist accomplished what the owners could not. First, he separated the animals, putting them in different rooms. Then, with each dog restrained by a leash, he gradually brought them closer, with reinforcement for gentle behavior. Conditioning worked. The dogs could once again coexist.

In another case, the owners' behavior shaped the dog's behavior. The dog, who had always been left alone in the house when his owners went to work, began to destroy household belongings when left alone. The psychologist's solution: Leave the house as usual, but return within five minutes; next time, return in fifteen minutes. The idea was to show the animal that it was never going to be left alone for very long. Whether or not the animal "got the idea," the destructive behavior stopped.

Behavior modification techniques may be used to train animals, but more notice is given their use in training humans. Self-modification, in particular, is increasingly in vogue. In self-modification you adopt the principle of operant conditioning to attack a problem behavior: excessive smoking or overeating or timidity. You do just what any behavior modifier would do: Pinpoint the particular behavior; keep track of its frequency; and select a reinforcement which will work for you.

The target behavior itself should be a manageable unit. Benjamin Franklin's program of self-modification might have been more successful if he had broken his idealized virtues into manageable components. He was aiming for temperance, which he defined as "eat not to dullness, drink not to elevation." It might have been easier, at least at first, to reinforce the specific behavior of eating smaller amounts at dinner.

Franklin was on the right track, however, in recording his failures. Behavior therapists recommend recordkeeping as an aid to awareness. Constant smokers or overeaters are often totally unaware of their behavior; writing it down every single time a cigarette or a morsel of food finds its way to their lips is a big step toward modifying the undesirable behavior. Sometimes additional steps are necessary; the chain smoker may not even be able to keep an accurate record unless something makes him realize that he's reached for a cigarette. Wrapping the cigarette package, so that it must be deliberately unwrapped before a cigarette can be reached, may produce the necessary awareness. It may also break the chain of conditioned response, interrupt the accustomed procedure.

If you want to combat overeating, too, an important step is self-monitoring, keeping track of when and what and where you eat. Most overeaters, the theory goes, eat automatically: They reach for snacks every time they walk through the kitchen, nibble while watching television, eat quickly at mealtimes, and then eat more while waiting for others to finish. They don't have to be hungry in order to eat; the conditioned stimulus of, for example, television will prompt the reach for food. And they're often not aware of just how often they eat. Keeping track is the first step toward awareness.

Then comes the hard part: cutting down. This involves unlearning the learned behavior of eating, detaching it from the stimuli that produce overeating. One method: Reduce the stimuli that prompt eating; limit eating only to an "eating place," a dining or restaurant table. Another method: Slow down; put your fork down between each bite. And another: Create a positive consequence for yourself every time you cut out an accustomed snack. Promise yourself a movie, for instance, or a new record if you manage to skip television-time nibbling for a whole week. Help yourself along by keeping your hands busy while you watch; take up needlework or work on a model airplane. Make yourself clean out your closet or do something else equally unappealing if you add another snack instead.

The same technique can work if you have other habits you would like to break. One teenager used self-modification to break his habit of excessive swearing. A high-school athlete who'd started swearing around the locker room, and used it at first as casually as most teens do, he found that it had got out of hand. He was jolted to this awareness when he lost his post as high-school representative to an interschool sports conference. Then, as reported in *How to Make and Break Habits*, a therapist suggested that he needed to stop himself before he started. The problem was stopping in time. The technique: a brightly colored paper-bag mask which he could hold to his face every time he started to swear. The combination of self-awareness imposed by the mask and the negative reinforcement of being laughed at by his friends did the trick; swearing was brought under control.

Self-modification can help you break habits; it can also be effective in establishing new habits. If you're having trouble buckling down to homework, for instance, you might set up a program of operant conditioning for yourself. Set a specific time for study, and tell your family you don't want to be disturbed. That part is easy. But you don't want to spend the allotted time staring into space. To keep your mind on business, put the kitchen timer to use: Set it for five minutes, and *study* for those five minutes; if your mind wanders, start again. At the end of five minutes, take a break for two minutes. Once you're regularly paying attention for the five minutes, increase the time periods; work up to an hour of study and a ten-minute break. If you're tempted to stop a little early, do one more problem or read two more pages.

Your sense of accomplishment plus the likelihood of improved grades should provide adequate reinforcement. If your parents have been after you to develop good study habits, however, they may be willing to add some additional reinforcement. Perhaps you can work out a point system. If you study, actually study, every evening for a whole week, you may be able to earn a special reward on the weekend. The reward will depend on your interests and, of course, on your parents. It could be anything from being excused from the Sunday dishwashing stint to having a riding lesson to the use of the family car.

The same techniques can be applied to all sorts of behavior, from being on time to keeping your room neat to smiling more often. They can be specifically applied to social behavior, to getting along with other people. Assertiveness training uses behavioral principles to show people how to take command of their lives, get over excessive shyness, and stand up for themselves. One of the techniques involves imagery, living through an experience in the mind so that it loses the terror it has in actuality. Take the specific behavior you are afraid to perform, psychologist Herbert Fensterheim recommends, and go through it in your mind, breaking it into small parts and imagining each part in detail. Select a pleasant thought as a reinforcer and imagine that thought at each step of the way. If, for instance, you are shy about talking to a certain classmate, you might picture a string of events in which you start a conversation, perhaps in the hall outside a classroom, with a comment about a teacher, then progress through a chat about the school's baseball team. As you picture each part of the conversation, you can reduce anxiety by switching to your mental image of something relaxing and pleasant—such as floating in a canoe or enjoying an ice cream sundae or listening to music. It will take some mental practice, and a change of attitude, say assertiveness training therapists, but you should be able to carry on the conversation in real life.

The key to assertiveness training, as to all forms of behavior modification, is self-understanding. You must identify in very specific terms the behavior you want to change and/or the behavior you want to acquire. You must keep accurate records of your behavior; maybe you don't become tongue-tied as often as you think you do. You should try to understand the entire chain of behavior, so that you can work on one part of it at a time. Try to control the stimuli that trigger your behavior: A new clock-radio may help you to get to school on time; rearranged closet space may help your neatness campaign. Reward yourself for performing the desired behavior, mentally and/or concretely. Set your standards higher and higher, so that the rewards are harder to earn. And let other people know what you are doing, so that they can provide reinforcement too.

Don't give up too soon. If you've picked a habit you can actually acquire, if you've selected appropriate reinforcements, if you've provided yourself with plenty of reminders, you can modify your behavior. And you won't have to explore your unconscious. In the psychoanalytic view, behavior problems are treated as a symptom of underlying conflict. In behaviorist terms, problems are treated as behavior . . . and behavior can be changed.

PART IV

Thought Styles

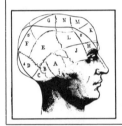

Jean Piaget:
A theory of the mind

Do you remember, when you were little, being asked to show off by counting to 100? Do you perhaps also remember not having the least idea what the numbers meant? When you were in the seventh grade, did your dad get upset because you just couldn't seem to grasp algebraic concepts? Did the same concepts suddenly become crystal clear a couple of years later? Now that you're in high school, are you appalled at all the misery in the world, determined that it's possible to end hunger and war and disease if only people would try? Do adults, parents and teachers, infuriate you by saying "You'll see, it's not that easy, you just don't know enough yet"?

In each case, according to the theories of the Swiss psychologist Jean Piaget, you have been demonstrating the style of thought, the kind of logic, appropriate to your stage of development. Children and adults think differently, Piaget has found. Indeed, children think differently at different ages. You weren't being stubborn when you couldn't set out eight apples for eight people after successfully counting to 100. You weren't dumb when you just couldn't get a handle on algebra. And you aren't being silly in thinking the problems of the world can be solved. It has nothing to do with quantitative knowledge, with the amount of information that's been pounded into your head. It has everything to do with the quality of thought, with the way in which you see things at a particular age. You don't respond to things in a different way, reach different conclusions from those of your parents and teachers, either because you are dumb or because you are lacking in experience. You reach different conclusions because you perceive the world in a unique way. It isn't more knowledge that will make you see things the way your parents do; it is growth, moving onward to a new mental stage.

Piaget's theories, these theories of sequential growth, have been developed through meticulous observation, not of large numbers of children but of a few children (notably his own three) over a long period of time. Actually, Piaget, who brought his own early training as a zoologist to the observations of children, was something of a child prodigy himself. His first scientific article, on a rare albino sparrow, was published when he was ten. His early teen years were devoted to the study of mollusks, under the guidance of a local museum director. In 1918, at the age of twenty-one, he completed his doctorate in the natural sciences. He then turned his attention to psychology, specifically the development of mental processes in children, and over the course of the decades has published some thirty books and innumerable articles. Not everyone agrees with Piaget's conclusions. But everyone does agree that Piaget's influence has been significant.

Piaget's theories

Piaget is not a behaviorist. He believes in the existence of internal mental responses, and his own findings have been to some extent intuitive. Piaget is also not a Freudian. He believes that the environment influences those internal mental responses. But he has been influenced by Freud's work. He has done for the mind, in fact, what Freud has done for the psyche: He has shown that the mind develops by stages, with each stage building on the one before. And he has shown that the processes of thought are governed both by maturation and by interaction with the environment.

Some of Piaget's technical terminology may look formidable, but the theory itself is not difficult to understand. Once you get past the hurdle of jargon, you will probably recognize much of what Piaget has to say. He defines intelligence, first of all, as adaptation to the environment. That adaptation takes place through the two processes he calls assimilation and accommodation, processes which interact throughout life in different ways as the individual meets the demands of the environment. When you assimilate new information, you fit it into the information you already possess, like a new piece into a jigsaw puzzle. When you accommodate to that new information, you modify the assumptions you already possess, in order to make room for the new information; you may, to continue the analogy, have to change the outer shape of the puzzle on which you are working.

A constant balance is maintained between assimilation and accommodation, through the process Piaget calls equilibration; this is a concept based on equilibrium or balance. You move, as you mature, from one level of thought process to another, through equilibration, through understanding a particular situation and applying the understanding to new situations.

Equilibration is essential. Without it you could not move from stage to stage. But it is not the only essential ingredient. Piaget also recognizes maturation, physical experience, and social interaction as vital to mental growth. Maturation implies biological growth, the acquisition of structures of mind which make more-advanced thought possible; a two-year-old, no matter what, cannot master calculus. Physical experience implies just that: the experience with concrete objects that enable you to understand what they are. Laboratory courses in the physical sciences are built on the premise that practice is as important as theory when it comes to comprehension. Social interaction refers to the exchange of ideas among people; in order to learn abstract concepts such as "roundness" and "fairness," a child must interact with other children, with parents, and with other adults.

One more bit of jargon: Piaget describes mental development in terms of operations, the way in which the individual makes sense of objects and events. In the earliest stages of mental development, operations must be concrete; the young child must be able to see and to touch if he is to understand. With maturity, the individual becomes capable of performing mental operations in terms of abstractions; thought and language take the place of physical contact.

Piaget's stages

The normal child, influenced by equilibration and maturation, physical experience and social interaction, moves through a series of cognitive stages. Each stage builds on the preceding stage; it is impossible to skip any stage. Some children may progress faster than others, some children will be slower, so all ages are approximate, but all children move through the sequence in order. See if you can recognize in these stages the characteristics of anyone you know: your younger brother or sister, a youngster for whom you may baby-sit, a classmate or friend.

The sensory-motor stage lasts from birth to about the age of two. It's hard to compare a helpless infant with a walking, talking, often rebellious two-year-old. But in Piaget's scheme of things, there's not that much difference. The unifying factor lies, of course, in mental process. During this entire period the child is governed by bodily interaction with the environment. At the beginning of this "prethought" period, in fact, the child cannot distinguish between himself and his environment. He is totally egocentric, totally involved in himself. He is, in Freudian terminology, dominated by the id. The toddler, later in this stage, may be walking around and may be distinguishing himself from other people and from objects, but he is still dominated by physical sensation, by the need to relate everything to his own person.

If you spend any time observing the behavior of babies in the sensory-motor stage, you will notice their tremendous self-absorption; you will also notice how quickly and how much they change. At the beginning, of course, infants don't do very much. But they learn remarkably quickly. The sucking reflex present at birth, for instance, is quickly modified by experience: A baby just a couple of weeks old will anticipate sucking at the sight of food. A very young baby will also try to repeat pleasant sensations, in what Piaget called circular reactions. The thumb may find its way to the mouth by accident the first time; repetition is deliberate. A swinging toy may make an interesting rattling noise; the baby will try to swing the toy again. (Behaviorists, of course, describe such actions as the result of conditioned learning. Behaviorists also imply that conditioning can be used to teach just about anything to just about anybody. Piaget insists that learning can take place only at the appropriate stage of mental development, in the appropriate sequence.)

By the middle of the first year, at the heart of what Freud described as the oral stage, the infant is reaching out to experience, picking up interesting objects whenever they are within reach, and frequently testing their taste as well as their texture. Later on in the first year, as the baby begins to get around on all fours, exploration of the surroundings becomes purposeful. If you take care of an eight- to twelve-month-old infant during his waking hours, you've probably noticed this intense curiosity about the environment. Such a baby will explore the entire household, dumping the contents of kitchen cabinets and wastebaskets with equal enthusiasm. One minute you may find him chewing on a pot handle, the next on a piece of cellophane.

A slightly older child, in the second year, will continue his explorations. But he is also beginning, just beginning, to use thought to solve problems, and to respond to verbal direction. With the onset of language, this child no longer needs to rely exclusively on physical sensation. If you put an active year-old baby down for a nap when he doesn't want to nap, he may struggle hard to climb out of his crib, trying one escape route after another. If you do the same thing with a child of twenty months or so, he will stop and think, then try an approach which has a chance of working.

But the most interesting development of this entire cognitive stage revolves around the concept of object permanence, the concept that objects have an independent existence. You know that your teacher exists even when you are at home and cannot see the teacher; you know that this book exists, occupies a position in space, whether or not you can see it. Infants, totally egocentric as they are, do not know this; objects exist for infants only when they are present and visible. The concept that objects are permanent develops gradually. You can watch the concept develop.

If you show a bright rattle to a young baby, capture his attention, then move the rattle within his field of vision, he will follow the toy with his eyes. Remove the rattle, however, and he won't even look for it. It has ceased to exist. By the time the baby is six months old, this is no longer so: Remove the rattle from view and he will keep on looking. But put the toy under a handkerchief and that's it; it has vanished, along with the baby's interest. At a year old, this same baby is a lot more sophisticated; he knows that things exist when they are hidden, and the game of peekaboo, as a result, becomes a lot of fun. But you can still play some tricks. Hide that shiny rattle under a handkerchief and the baby will gleefully reach for it. Hide it again, under a second handkerchief, and the baby will look for it under the first—even if he has seen you place it under the second cloth and even if its outline is clearly visible. Object permanence, at a year, goes only so far.

Children under the age of about two, in Piaget's view, are dominated by physical sensation. They live very much in the present; both mentally and emotionally they are tied to immediate events. If the telephone rings just as a toddler falls and bangs his knee, for instance, he may associate the telephone ringing with his accident. If mother puts on a coat and the child has seen mother leave him with a sitter after putting on her coat in the past, he may know she is leaving him again. And with his immature concept of object permanence, he may not be at all sure that she is coming back; he may not even be quite sure that she exists when out of his sight. The end of the sensory-motor stage is marked by the development of the concept of object permanence and by the beginning of the ability to substitute symbols for the concrete.

The preoperational stage begins, at two or two and a half, as the child begins to develop ways of representing objects and events through symbols, including the symbol of language. This is a highly significant step, because only through symbols can you visualize things that are not present; only through symbols can you solve problems.

The abstract capabilities of preschool children are, of course, severely limited. For one thing, children from two to seven are still, by and large, egocentric. They know at this stage that people and objects outside themselves have an independent existence. But they conceive of that existence only in relationship to themselves. A good example is the preschooler who covers her eyes and insists that you can't see her. And, for another thing, the verbal ability of small children often masks an inability to deal with abstractions. Young children are very literal-minded: Told about a planned family flight to Europe, one three-year-old, who had seen lots of airplanes, tearfully told his parents that he couldn't go because he didn't know how to fly yet. Told that someone had "died laughing," a five-year-old saw a macabre image.

Piaget conducted many experiments with the style of preoperational thought. He determined that children at this stage, although they can use language and understand some concepts, are still bound by perception, by what they can actually see. They do not see transformation, the process of change. They see life as a series of still pictures instead of as a moving picture. Show a five-year-old a rod or stick in a vertical position and let it fall to the tabletop. The child, asked to draw what he sees, will picture the rod in its first position and its last, but not in between. Because preoperational children do not see transformation, they have particular trouble with classification and with conservation.

Classification is the ability to categorize objects, particularly when the objects fall into both a small group and a larger one. Pennies, for instance, are both pennies and coins. A preschooler who can tell you quite correctly that there are more pennies than nickels in a handful of coins will probably not be able to tell you accurately whether there are more pennies or coins. He will simply be unable to sort out these overlapping categories. He may also insist that it is impossible to be two things at once, as did the youngster (quoted by David Elkind, an American psychologist who has studied with Piaget) who insisted that he could not be both Protestant and American at the same time—unless, of course, he moved.

Conservation is the ability to recognize that the basic attributes of an object remain the same even if the object changes in appearance. If that sounds complicated, think of a lump of clay. If you take two lumps of equal size and mold them into similarly shaped balls, both you and the preschooler will know that the lumps of clay are identical. If you then flatten one of the two balls, or roll it into a snake, you will still know that the lumps of clay are the same size. The preschooler, limited to preoperational thought, to what he can actually see, will not. He will guess, more likely than not, that the longer piece of clay is the larger.

Similarly, if you take a cup of water and pour it first into a tall, thin container and then into a short, fat container, you will know that the amount of liquid remains the same; it still measures one cup. The preschool child, even though he has watched the experiment, will probably insist that there is more water in the taller container.

Conservation also applies to number. Preoperational children may be very glib when it comes to counting, but this does not mean that they understand the concept of number. Any number of experiments can be devised to bear this out. Arrange checkers in two rows of equal length, for example, and ask a young child to count the rows and agree that there is the same number in each row. Then, while the child watches, stretch one row out or bunch it up. The child will now insist, even if he has watched you move the checkers and even if he counts the rows again, that one row contains more than the other. The dimension of space means more than the concept of number.

The preoperational child cannot focus on more than one aspect of something at a time. If the lump of clay appears longer, it must be bigger. If the water level is higher, even though the glass is thinner, there must be more water. The preoperational child also cannot comprehend that some things are reversible, that a lump of clay can assume one shape and then another, that a group of checkers can be stretched or compressed and yet remain the same, or that if 8 plus 4 equals 12, then 12 minus 4 must equal 8.

The preoperational stage lasts until age seven or even a little beyond, and since the ability to classify and the ability to conserve are essential to success in school, especially in mathematics, it is little wonder that some children confront nothing but frustration in the early grades. If Piaget is right, and many educators think he is, then learning in these early grades should take place largely through concrete objects which children can manipulate—blocks and counting rods and the like. With such teaching aids, young children are better able to learn. When they are better able to learn, behavior problems are less likely to result.

The stage of concrete operations is reached, at about age seven, when a child begins to think logically and not just intuitively. The child at this stage is no longer limited to what he sees and what he does. He can understand that the lumps of clay remain the same even though they look different. By the time he is ten or eleven he can apply this understanding to more complex problems involving weight and volume. He can think through a problem. If the young child misplaces a toy, he may wander through the entire house looking for it; if the school-age child misplaces a toy, he is more likely to think back to where he has been and where he might have left the toy, and then look for it.

But the child in this stage, from seven to about eleven, is still not an adult. Thought processes, although far more advanced and far more capable of symbols and abstraction than at earlier ages, are still tied, for the most part, to the concrete. Show a group of eight-year-olds three wooden rods and they will understand, nodding their heads as you demonstrate, that rod A is longer than rod C and that rod C is longer than rod B; therefore, they willingly agree, rod A is the longest of all. Give them a similar problem in verbal terms—Ann is taller than Carol and Carol is taller than Betty—and confusion reigns; the child in this stage of development cannot tell you who is the tallest. True hypothetical thought, the ability to reason "if thus, then so," does not appear until the adolescent years. By now, you can easily tell that Ann is the tallest of the three girls.

Because of this remaining link to the concrete, children in the elementary-school years often have difficulty with hypothetical situations. Sixth-graders, on the verge of formal thought at the age of eleven or twelve, may be delighted at the challenge of creating a kingdom peopled by two-inch-high humans; they will go to great lengths to devise settings and situations scaled to this size. Younger children, still tied to concrete operations, may flatly refuse the assignment; if there is no such thing as two-inch-high humans, then there can be no kingdom.

Children in the middle years have shed some of their egocentricity. They understand that other people have an independent existence, and they can get along with other people in ways that preschoolers can not. Very young children become increasingly involved with groups of friends. Games, with their rules and rituals, are very important to children in this stage, because they fulfill a sense of order and define a way of relating to others.

The stage of formal operations, the stage that begins at about the age of twelve and corresponds with the junior- and senior-high-school years, is the point at which most young people approach true logical thought. Some people, of course, including some adults, never do reach this level. Some people will always comprehend information more readily if it is presented in a concrete way.

Some educators believe that this need not be so, that for-

jective abilities. But how you feel about those abilities, your perception of yourself, is at least as important as the qualities themselves. How you feel about your abilities determines what you do with them. You may know that your measured IQ is higher than average, Don Hamachek of Michigan State University points out, but without the self-confidence and faith in yourself to act on that knowledge, the IQ itself is useless. If you've somehow been convinced that you're dumb, perhaps through endless comparisons with an older brother or sister or cousin, then paper scores on paper tests won't help. If, on the contrary, no matter what your measured IQ, you've always been treated as a person of value, a person with something to contribute, your self-respect will be intact.

Newborn infants have no sense of self. That sense takes root gradually as the infant becomes aware of his ability to influence and control the environment in specific ways. Each time a rattle is successfully grasped, a step successfully taken, the child's sense of competence is enhanced. The sense of self grows as the child becomes increasingly aware of his separateness, his uniqueness. The infant realizes that the image in the mirror is his own. The preschooler is consulted about what he would like for dinner. And the sense of self matures as the child, secure in his world, knows that he belongs.

This, of course, is the ideal sequence. Not every child grows up in circumstances which permit the development of a secure sense of self. Humanists hold nonetheless that every person is intrinsically a person of value, that every human being has worth. Humanist psychologists believe that human nature is basically good.

Unlike Freudian psychoanalysts, humanist psychologists take an optimistic and hopeful view of human nature. The self-selected goals are generally positive goals, the theory goes, as each individual strives to develop his or her own po-

mal reasoning can be taught; others, adhering more closely to Piaget's position, believe that experience helps but that maturation is at least as important. Those who believe that students can be helped to move from one stage to the next have developed specific curricula in some subjects, curricula designed to help students make the transition to formal operations. Laboratory programs in biology and physics, for instance, relate the concrete to the abstract.

Those adolescents who have reached the level of formal operations can reason scientifically, weigh ideas one against the other, think in hypothetical terms, and solve many different types of problems through logical abstract thought. "An adolescent, unlike the child," Piaget has written, "is an individual who thinks beyond the present and forms theories about everything, delighting especially in consideration of that which is not." An adolescent, engrossed in the world of ideas, can think about his own thoughts. At this stage you can argue the merits of various systems of government, figure out the best way to tackle an experiment in chemistry, appreciate the subtlety of a political cartoon, discuss religious philosophy, and write an imaginative essay based on the premise that cats can fly. You can visualize colonies in space, and a perfect political system on Earth. You can think beyond the realities of the present into the possibilities of the future.

You have reached this point through building on each of the preceding stages. As one psychologist, Mary Ann Spencer Pulaski, has put it: "The young child can deal with concrete objects; the schoolchild can deal with them in thought; the adolescent is freed from the bonds of physical reality to soar into the realm of hypothetical possibilities."

But this level of achievement does not mean that mental growth is complete. Not just yet. Adolescents, Piaget found, are still egocentric, logical but not necessarily realistic. With the power to reason logically, to think in terms of the ideal, it may seem possible, even easy, to solve the problems of the world. Some adolescents, frustrated by what they see as adult unwillingness to work on the problems, turn to political activism; others retreat into dreamy idealism. With time, however, and with the reaching of the equilibrium that results from a balance between assimilation and accommodation, idealism is usually tempered by reality.

Piaget emphasizes the course of cognitive growth. He does not deal with personality or with motivation, with why you have a love-hate relationship with your brother or why you are afraid of dogs. But he does deal with an important aspect of human behavior: how we think and how we learn to think. His ideas have found increasing acceptance in recent years. "Sesame Street," the popular children's television program, is based on his theories. So are a number of innovative classrooms, particularly those in which learning is based on self-discovery. If you are the initiator of your own learning, according to Jean Piaget, you will learn far more. And you will advance to succeeding levels of thought, to an increasingly more sophisticated ability to reason.

PART V

Humanism: Psychology of the Self

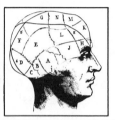

Self-actualization and self-fulfillment

Humanism is the third major force in psychology today. As its name implies, humanism concentrates not on biological drives or on environmental forces but on what is most human about human beings: the individual human self. Humanism defines the self, the inner core of a person as perceived by that person, as the most important element in personality. Humanist theory describes how the self develops, through self-understanding, conscious motivation, and self-fulfillment based on self-selected goals. Humanism in practice, as the next chapter will show, works toward helping people develop the positive self-image that makes self-fulfillment possible.

Self-perception—the self-image—is a vital part of the equation. Self-perception, how you feel about yourself, actually governs behavior. You have certain qualities, certain ob-

tential to the fullest. You want to be the best person you possibly can, in short, to develop your own unique attributes.

Where Freud stressed unconscious motivation and biological drives which must be overcome in order to achieve mental health, moreover, humanists stress that motivation is conscious and that the natural drive is for the attainable goal of self-fulfillment. Where Freud was concerned with the causes of emotional disturbance, humanists are interested in healthy normal human beings and with what makes them that way. "To oversimplify the matter somewhat," humanist psychologist Abraham Maslow has written, "it is as if Freud supplied to us the sick half of psychology and we must now fill it out with the healthy half."

Unlike the behaviorist psychologists, too, humanists believe that human beings are creatures of free will, in charge of their own destiny. "The potential to learn and the power to act lie within the person," humanist Carl Rogers has written, "rather than in an expert dealing with him or her, or in a system controlling him or her." Human beings must interact with the environment and with other people, but they are not shaped and conditioned by those forces. Instead, each individual reacts to experiences with others in a special, subjective way. This personal quality of experience, akin to self-perception, is very important in humanist theory.

Humanism is a significant force in contemporary psychology precisely because of these two factors: It states that you, yourself, are important. And it puts you in charge of your own destiny. Humanist psychology, what some have called the psychology of self-fulfillment, has had a profound impact on our society, on literature, on education, and on the way we view ourselves. This impact is visible in our vocabulary, in the proliferation of words involving the way we view ourselves: *self-confidence, self-esteem, self-concept, self-image.*

There are many humanist psychologists. There are two

men, however, whose names are virtually synonymous with humanism: Abraham Maslow and Carl Rogers.

Abraham Maslow

Maslow, who has been called the father of humanist psychology, is a twentieth-century theoretician; born in 1908, he died in 1970. His theory, based on his study of forty-nine outstanding people, past and present, is a theory of growth. How, Maslow wondered, did creative people get to be that way? How did they find self-fulfillment? How did they become models for other human beings?

Maslow began his study with two greatly admired teachers. Seeing them as distinct individuals, he nonetheless found a common thread, an exciting clue to human creativity. He extended his study to include other people whom he subjectively judged as strong and creative, and developed a description of what he then called self-actualized people. Self-actualized people, as Maslow describes them, are the most fully human of human beings. They use and exploit all of their abilities, capacities, and talents. They fulfill themselves, while doing the best that they can possibly do. They—such people as Abraham Lincoln and Eleanor Roosevelt—live to the fullest.

Self-actualized people, furthermore, display specific traits. They accept themselves, other people, and nature, without anxiety and without much concern. They are more interested in problem solving than in self-analysis. They show spontaneity, and both appreciate and demonstrate rich emotional reactions. They are independent and like solitude and privacy—Maslow calls them "self-sufficient and self-contained"—but identify with the human species and experience deep interpersonal relationships. They perceive reality accurately and don't indulge in wishful thinking. They are creative. They are ethical. They are open to new experience, information, and ideas. And they, more than most people,

92

have what Maslow calls peak experiences, the ecstatic sensation associated with sudden insight and/or fulfilled creativity.

Maslow, for whom self-actualization is the built-in drive toward a healthy personality, defines self-actualization as something akin to creativity. He describes it as "experiencing fully, vividly, selflessly, with full concentration and total absorption. . . . At this moment of experiencing, the person is wholly and fully human."

This quality of being fully human is not limited to those narrowly defined as "creative." Maslow's concept is far broader. Sculptors and musicians do not have an exclusive claim to Maslow's brand of creativity. Self-actualized, creative people are those people in any field—housewives or students, athletes or carpenters or psychiatrists—who have the ability to see and the willingness to say that the emperor has no clothes. They are people with a fresh outlook, people who feel free to express their thoughts and feelings. They retain, in fact, what Maslow calls a childlike (not childish) spontaneity and expressiveness.

Not very many people are fully self-actualized. But the key aspect of Maslow's theory is that it is a theory of growth. It describes human development in terms of growth toward a self-actualized state. Maslow, along with other humanist psychologists, holds that human beings have an inborn need to grow, to develop competence, and to move toward self-actualization. Self-actualization, in fact, may more accurately be called self-actualiz*ing;* it is a process of becoming rather than a state of being.

Young people move toward self-actualization just as adults do. In contrast to Freudian theory, which holds that growth is a process of struggle within the individual, Maslow believes that "healthy children *enjoy* growing and moving forward, gaining new skills, capacities and powers." Healthy children are eager to grow up, to mature, to develop their abilities to the fullest.

But self-actualization is not possible, in children or in adults, unless and until basic human needs are met. The hierarchy of basic human needs starts with the physical and moves through the emotional. The most primary need is for the satisfaction of hunger and thirst; a hungry person finds it difficult, if not impossible, to be creative or to think of self-fulfillment. Next in the hierarchy is the need for safety. This is both a physical and a psychological need. People must be physically secure and they must be psychologically comfortable, free from both types of fear, before they can move onward toward self-actualization.

The other needs are also important. You must feel that you belong, that people care about you, before you can develop further; this is sometimes called a need for love. You must also feel confident in your own abilities, with self-esteem based on recognition of those abilities. And last, highest in the hierarchy, is the need for self-actualization itself. This need, most difficult to satisfy, is the need to reach one's potential; it can be recognized only when all the other needs have been met.

There is a constant progression through the hierarchy. The satisfaction of one need leads to the urge to satisfy another need. "The organism is dominated and its behavior organized," Maslow has written, "only by unsatisfied needs." Translated, this implies that only those who are both physically and emotionally secure, loved, and self-confident can become fully functioning, self-actualized human beings. Only these people are fully open to peak experiences. Psychologically healthy human beings, however, are all those who have moved beyond the lowest level of needs, those who, even if not yet self-actualized, are concerned with the enhancement of life. These are people who, if not self-actualized, are self-actualizing. They are moving toward full humanity, toward becoming all that it is possible for them to become.

Carl Rogers

Maslow studied psychologically healthy individuals to develop his theory of self-actualization. Carl Rogers, a contemporary of Maslow's, has studied people in therapy to develop his theory of the fully functioning human being. He revolutionized the role of the therapist, and therapy itself, in fact, by participating in the expression of feelings. In contrast to the father-figure Freudian psychoanalyst, who offers explanations and interpretations if he speaks at all, the Rogerian therapist offers understanding and acceptance. The result has been called person-centered or client-centered therapy.

In client-centered therapy, the therapist enters what Rogers calls an "intensely personal and subjective relationship" with the client. It is a person-to-person relationship, in which the therapist accepts the client as a person of value. It is a relationship in which the therapist empathizes with the client, putting himself in the client's position so that full sympathy and support can be offered. And it is a relationship in which the therapist, instead of offering solutions to problems or even guidelines to solutions, is interested solely in helping the client to be himself.

The client-centered therapist must be genuinely interested in the client and genuinely accepting of the client's feelings. Then the client, as he finds that his thoughts and feelings can be expressed without fear of criticism, moves toward self-acceptance. As clients begin to like and accept themselves, they become more capable of sharing relationships with other people.

Client-centered therapy began and still exists as the traditional two-person procedure. In the 1960s, however, the emphasis shifted. Group therapy became increasingly popular. And groups, sometimes called encounter or sensitivity groups, began to attract people who would not necessarily have sought therapy, people who simply wanted to move toward greater self-acceptance. Today, in what many observers see as a reaction to increasing dehumanization in society as a whole, there are groups of many different kinds, under various kinds of leadership.

In Rogerian groups, as in client-centered individual practice, the therapist (in groups he is often called a facilitator) offers support and understanding rather than direction. The group itself, unless convened for a particular purpose (as for instance in a drug-abuse program), takes its own direction. Whatever it decides, however, the emerging relationship among the group members dominates the proceedings. Rogers sees the rapid spread of groups, in fact, as an expression of hunger for "relationships which are close and real; in which feelings and emotions can be spontaneously expressed without first being carefully censored or bottled up. . . ." He sees encounter groups themselves as an opportunity for more and more people to shed their masks, to reveal the private self in addition to the public self. This revelation, whether it comes in one-to-one client-centered therapy or in group encounter, is the first step toward becoming fully functioning, fully human.

Rogers observed men and women, in individual therapy and in group encounter, as they progressed toward mental health, toward self-acceptance. He analyzed the characteristics they exhibited in the process and developed his definition of the fully functioning human being. The fully functioning person, he decided, rather like Maslow's self-actualized individual, accepts his feelings and expresses them openly. He just as willingly accepts the feelings of others. He listens to others, really listens, and encourages others to express their feelings. He is confident enough of himself, secure in his self-esteem, so as not to be threatened either by his own feelings or by the feelings of others. He can both accept and give love, without guilt and without anxiety. He is satisfied, nonetheless, to meet his own expectations rather than those of others. He gets along well with other people, lives fully in the present, and is open to new ideas. He has the ability and the willingness to make independent decisions. He is also creative. "With his sensitive openness to the world, his trust of his own ability to form new relationships with the environment," Rogers has written, "he would be the type of person from whom creative products and creative living emerge."

Rogers sums up the above characteristics and defines the fully functioning person, the ideal end-point of psychological growth, in terms of three dominant traits: This person is an individual fully open to his own experiences, without defense mechanisms to shut out experience. He allows experience to shape his personality, thereby becoming somewhat unpredictable but remaining open to growth. And, above all, he trusts in his own self, in his own ability to feel what is right and to do what is right.

This trust in the self is basic to Rogers's thought. In the broadest terms, it means a trust in human beings, "a basic trust in constructive potential of the person." In specific terms, it means your own trust in yourself. You often face situations in which you can rely either on the opinion of others or on your own best judgment. Should you take a particular history course, known to be interesting but tough? Should you go out with a certain person? Should you take another drink? If you are a fully functioning person, you will make your decision and base your behavior on your own experiences, feelings, and sense of what is right for you.

This, of course, is difficult to do. It is difficult for most adults. And it is doubly difficult for young people in the school years. Your self is not that well established, not yet that familiar to you, that you can rely on it without hesitation. But Rogers's notion, like Maslow's, is that the personality (at any age) is not static. The psychologically healthy personality is always growing, always changing. And the healthiest of all is the individual who is moving toward the status of being fully functioning.

Rogers uses a computer analogy to further define the state of being fully functioning. The fully functioning person is like a "giant electronic computing machine," absorbing and processing data from all the senses, from memory, from previous learning, and from all the internal and external states of being. He shuts nothing out. He lives completely in the present because, with all this "input," he is totally aware of each moment. And—he does not really exist. The fully functioning personality, Rogers has been careful to point out, is a goal rather than a reality. It is a state, like that of being self-actualized, which is a desirable target. It is a state which is occasionally attained by some people.

You can move toward this ideal state by being open to experience, by being willing to take some emotional risks, by being flexible and willing to change. The neurotic person is characterized by rigidity, by a self-image so fragile that change is threatening. The psychologically healthy individual, in contrast, is characterized by continual growth. Growth, in turn, is marked by the willingness to take risks. Thus, it goes hand in hand with an openness to new experience.

Risks, on an emotional level, are different for different people. It can be emotionally threatening for some people to speak up in class. It can be emotionally risky for a great many people to admit strong feelings of affection. It can be easy to say "I love you" in tender moments, but hard to say "Hey, I really like you" to a friend or a brother. Taking the risk may result in some hurt. But the end result, in Rogers's view, is a person living to full potential. This, he feels, is a goal worth some risk.

Criticism of humanist psychology
It can be hard to disagree with advocates of self-fulfillment. But humanism does have its critics. There are four main points of contention: Humanism is unscientific. Humanism is

a romantic, unrealistic theory. Humanism has led to a selfish emphasis on the individual at the expense of society. Humanist encounter groups have been more destructive than constructive. Let's look at the criticisms one by one.

The first, that humanism is too vague to be scientific, is tied to the humanist emphasis on subjective interpretation of experience. How can you tell if you're having a peak experience? How can you, or anyone else, know if you are self-actualizing or fully functioning? What kind of objective evaluation is possible?

The next, that humanism is a superromantic, unworkable theory, is a matter of belief. There are many people who find it difficult to believe in the basic goodness of human nature. There are simply too many examples of human inhumanity, from world war to child abuse, to justify such belief. Humanists counter such arguments by pointing to environmental circumstances. It may be understandable for underemployed and emotionally deprived parents to take out their frustrations on their children. Improve the circumstances, help these people to become fully functioning human beings, and positive elements of human nature will triumph.

The emphasis on selfish individualism at the expense of society is another matter. Social critics have commented increasingly in recent years on the growing "me" orientation in our society. Some people point to the humanist emphasis on self-fulfillment, on discovering and fulfilling one's own potential, as the root cause for all manner of social change, from the rising numbers of women in the work force to the rising rate of divorce. But humanists point out that self-understanding is just the first step to better human relationships, that accepting and expressing one's own feelings helps in accepting other people's feelings.

The last charge concerns the wildly proliferating encounter groups. It has several aspects. For one thing, although a group is supposed to find its own direction, the leader, or facilitator, does set the tone. Some facilitators are well trained. Others are not. Some are truly dedicated to helping the people in the group express their own feelings. Others have a particular goal in mind, a particular philosophy they are seeking to implement. Some use only verbal discussion. Others stress the importance of physical touch, of nonverbal communication.

For another, there is some question about whether the encounter experience, even if it is a good one, has any lasting effect. Do people who start to share their inner feelings in the supportive atmosphere of the group find acceptance or ridicule when they do the same thing at home or on the job? Do they start to become fully functioning? Or do they retreat to the same old patterns of thought and behavior? Does the encounter experience cement or shatter existing relationships?

And a third, more serious attack on encounter groups comes from those who charge that they can trigger psychotic breakdowns in people who are sensitive to attack. The groups operate on the theory that it is good to express feelings, whether those feelings are positive or negative. Some participants react well, even to negative feelings from others, and experience psychological growth. Others, perhaps more vulnerable to begin with, cannot take the strain. Rogers himself mentions reports of occasional psychotic episodes. He also refers to people who have turned to therapy to work through the painful feelings aroused but unresolved by the encounter experience. Such need for therapy may be a negative result of the encounter, or it may be positive, helping the individual to move still further toward the goal of becoming fully functioning.

Many of these criticisms, made by reputable people, are valid at least to some degree. Yet humanism nonetheless has its appeal. It is, after all, a fundamentally optimistic view.

Both Maslow and Rogers hold that the inner nature of human beings is basically good. Both focus on human possibilities rather than human deficiencies. Both stress that a person, in Rogers's words, is "an emerging process, not a static end product."

This is a point of view which gives you some responsibility for yourself. The outer world still plays a role. The experiences you have at home, at school, and with your friends will inevitably affect both the way in which your self develops and your own perception of your self. Impossible standards set by parents can tarnish your self-image. A lack of popularity in school can damage your self-confidence.

But successful, self-confident people fail in some things. No one excels in every area. Perfection, both Maslow and Rogers admit, is not the goal. Improvement is. You, say the humanists, play the leading role in the drama of your own life. You can strive toward psychological growth, toward self-fulfillment, toward self-acceptance. Remind yourself that, as Carl Rogers put it, "I am someone, I am someone worth being, I am committed to being myself."

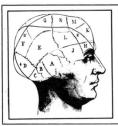

Humanism applied

Humanist psychology, like psychoanalysis and behaviorism, has spilled over from academic theory into everyday life. It was applied initially, through client-centered therapy, to the solution of individual problems. It has resulted, more or less directly, in the ever growing number of encounter and sensitivity groups through which people are "getting in touch" with their own feelings.

Participation in both client-centered therapy and encounter groups is elected, deliberately chosen. But humanism also affects you, on two fronts: It has had some impact on popular ideas about child rearing. And it has had a direct influence on contemporary education.

Humanism at home
Respect for the individual and for the feelings of the individ-

ual lies at the heart of humanist psychology. Parents have always demanded respect. Children, too, in the humanist view, deserve respect. When a child is respected as an individual, he or she can develop a secure sense of self and be able to move toward self-fulfillment.

The development of the self is paramount. Parents who have taken the advice of humanist psychologists are concerned with helping their children develop self-esteem. They make every effort to listen to their children's point of view, to convey the belief that children's points of view are worth hearing. They consult their children. At the same time, such parents respect themselves. Humanists have been accused of overpermissiveness, but it should be noted that their ideal home is not a child-centered home, not a home in which the child says "Jump" and the parent jumps. It is, instead, what Carl Rogers calls a person-centered home, a home in which every member of the family, of every age, is respected as a human being. In the person-centered home, Rogers says, "The child is treated as a unique person, worthy of respect, possessing the right to evaluate his experience in his own way, with wide powers of autonomous choice. The parent respects himself also, with rights which cannot be overridden by the child."

Mutual respect between parent and child sounds ideal. So does open communication between the generations, with honest expression and acceptance of feelings. It isn't, of course, that easy. Parents have good intentions, but very little training in the job of being parents. Parents also feel responsible for their children. The popular literature, therefore, is full of advice to parents on child guidance. Some of it tells parents how to mold their children, shape their behavior. Humanist psychologists, however, have developed specific techniques which can help parents and children communicate, get along, and respect each other as human beings.

the other person's behavior makes you feel. Parents who use I-messages don't tell their children how lazy and irresponsible the children are for leaving food-hardened dishes in the sink. Instead, they explain that they, the parents, feel discouraged at the sight of a messy kitchen after they've worked to keep it clean. If your eagerness for dinner is an indication of a wish to get out and join your friends, instead of a simple expression of hunger, your mother might send an I-message expressing her hurt.

I-messages, properly given, express real feelings. They require a willingness to express those primary feelings, rather than secondary or peripheral feelings. If you come home from a party at one-thirty in the morning when you had promised to be home by midnight, you may be greeted by an angry parent. The parent who is using an I-message will say that he is angry, not that you are terrible. But the parent who is really using the technique correctly, the one who is expressing primary feelings, will let you know first how relieved he is that you're home safely. His anger grew out of fear. You, in turn, realizing his concern, are more likely to be sorry that you are late. If all your parent expresses is anger, you may simply become defensive.

Mutual problem solving, the third step, is applied when the problem concerns you both. It grows out of Active Listening and the sending of I-messages. Mutual problem solving is what Gordon calls the No-lose Method, or Method III. Method I takes place when the parent (or teacher or boss) is dictatorial and wins every argument on the basis of sheer power. Method II takes place when the parent gives in and the child wins. Method III, the No-lose Method, takes place when mutual problem solving occurs and a mutually acceptable solution is found. Gordon believes that Method III can be used for most kinds of family disputes, with children of any age. Even toddlers, with limited verbal skills, react positively to Method III. Even toddlers can share in developing the solution to a mutual problem.

Method III relies on the humanist principle that each individual, a child as much as an adult, is worthy of respect. It applies to the parent-child relationship the same kinds of problem-solving approaches that might be used between spouses or friends. Your mother might be upset at your continual failure to clean your room. You can't see what all the fuss is about. Your mother could use Method I and order you to clean up the mess, on pain of being grounded. She could use Method II and throw up her hands in despair. Or she could talk it over with you and try to reach a mutually agreeable solution. In one family, such a solution involves simply keeping the teenager's door closed. In another, it involves trading chores: The mother cleans her teenage son's room in exchange for the son's cooking dinner a couple of evenings a week. If the son likes to cook, and chooses this solution, he will be motivated to stick to the bargain. Self-motivation, you will recall, is an important humanist concept. Self-respect is another. When people are treated with respect, solutions are possible. No one has to lose.

If you want to try the No-lose Method, however, you have to be willing to spend some time at problem solving. You also have to enlist the cooperation of your parents. Then, together, you can follow these steps: Identify the conflict, in terms of how it makes each party feel; generate possible solutions, as many as possible; evaluate the alternative solutions, eliminating those unacceptable to either side; decide on the best solution by testing it against your feelings; implement the decision; and, last, follow up with an evaluation of whether or not the solution is working. You'll find that with Active Listening and I-messages, with the recognition that your antagonist is a human being with legitimate feelings, most conflicts can be solved.

Humanism in the schools

The humanist philosophy shows up in the schools in a number of ways. One such way is through Teacher Effectiveness Training, a parallel to Parent Effectiveness Training. In T.E.T. teachers learn how to apply the techniques of Active Listening, I-messages, and mutual problem solving. In T.E.T. teachers lend a sympathetic, nonjudgmental ear to students' feelings, transmit their own strong feelings, and involve students in setting the rules for classroom behavior.

Another application of humanism is found in values clarification, a technique used in teaching students to formulate and recognize their own values. The heart of values clarification, and its link to humanism, lies in its assumption that children must be respected as individuals who can make a choice among values and who are free to express their own values. Choice by the child, involvement of the child, and respect for the child are key elements.

Values clarification, based on work by Louis E. Raths and Sidney B. Simon, is a specific attempt to get educators to move away from concentration on academic development and toward awareness of the whole child. Teachers trained in values clarification techniques encourage children to make choices and to make them freely, without coercion, either direct or subtle. They help students discover and examine available alternatives, and weigh the consequences of each alternative. They encourage children to consider just what it is that they prize and cherish. They give them opportunities to demonstrate their choices. And they encourage their students to act, behave, and live in accordance with the choices they have expressed.

Values clarification echoes the humanist emphasis on process. Values are not fixed, permanent and immutable, and imposed from outside. They are fluid, often changing, and developed from within. It is the valuing process that teachers can and should teach, not values themselves. Values clarification also echoes the humanist emphasis on involvement of the student. "Why must teachers see their role only as putting things into the mind of the child?" ask Raths and his colleagues in their book, *Values and Teaching*. Why can't teachers instead help a child define and organize what is already in his mind? Why can't teachers guide students in the process of selecting values?

Teacher training does not always deal with questions of values. Indeed, some school administrators, and some parents, question whether schools should get involved in questions of values at all. But advocates of values clarification point out that teachers transmit their own personal values, whether or not they set out to do so, in everything they say and do. Better, they suggest, to consciously help students develop their own values, their own expression of worth as human beings. There are specific techniques which can help.

One such technique is called the clarifying response. This is simply a device, like Active Listening, which puts the burden of working out feelings on the student. With a clarifying response the teacher avoids making judgments or evaluations. Instead, she tries, through a noncommittal remark or question, to make the student clarify his own response to a situation. For example: A student mentions that he is going on a weekend trip with his family. The teacher might say, "How nice," or "Have a good time." Or the teacher, trained in values clarification, might say, "Are you glad you're going?" The intent is not to provoke a discussion on the merits of family trips. The intent is simply to set the student thinking.

Another technique is the value continuum, symbolized by a horizontal line drawn between two extreme positions. "Where," the teacher asks, "would you place yourself on the line? Are you spend-it-all Charlie or save-it-all Sue? Or are you somewhere in between? Where?" The point of this exercise, whether applied to political issues or social issues or ethical issues, is that there are a variety of positions possible on any given issue. The point is that the individual must think through his own position.

There are other specific valuing techniques, to be used by groups or by individuals, in school or at home. But values clarification and Teacher Effectiveness Training, although both are rooted in humanist respect for the individual, are specific techniques applied to specific ends. The fullest application of humanist psychology in the schools, the application that focuses in equal measure on emotional well-being and on self-motivated learning, may be found in what is called open education, in the open classrooms and alternative schools taking root across the United States.

Open classrooms are most often found on the elementary level. They are based on Rogers's theories of self-directed learning plus Piaget's theories of cognitive development. The child at a particular stage of mental development, the theory goes, will eagerly learn all that he or she is capable of learning. He will learn the most through direct hands-on experience, through personal involvement and exploration and manipulation of materials. The teacher, therefore, does not need to "teach." Instead, the teacher acts, in Rogers's word, as a facilitator, guiding the students in their self-directed learning and providing opportunities for learning through exploration. Facilitators of learning in the open classroom do occasionally provide group instruction. More often they work with individual students, listening to reports on work accomplished, answering questions or asking them, offering advice or suggestions. The teacher is very much present, but acts as a catalyst, a spur to learning, rather than as a source of all knowledge and authority. He acts, in one description, as a travel agent, helping the student get where he wants to go in the best possible way.

In practical terms, open classrooms in the United States

were modeled after the British Infant School, an early-primary-grade setting for self-directed learning. The room itself, sometimes a corridor lined with classrooms, is likely to contain movable furniture, arranged in activity or interest centers of one kind and another. There will be a science corner, full of apparatus for exploration. How much water, students might wonder, is lost from a leaky faucet? In the science corner they can figure out how to find out. There will be a math corner, with measuring and counting devices of all kinds. How do you measure the brain capacity of a bird or rabbit, working solely from the animal's skull? There will be a reading corner, where youngsters will be found at any time of the school day, lying on the floor or curled up in a comfortable chair with a book.

Time is the important concept. More important than flexible space is flexible time. Children can move from activity to activity as they choose, and as interest dictates. A school-wide bell or a teacher's commands will not interrupt a science experiment on the verge of completion or a committee's lively discussion of a social studies project. There is great spillover, in any case, from subject to subject. A student fascinated by birds may construct models, draw pictures, write stories or poems, and look up reference books to back up observation and find out more. When groups of students work on such a project, sparked by their own curiosity, each one brings to the project and takes from it whatever means most to him.

Alternative schools are also centers for self-directed learning based on humanist psychology. Because they occur most often at the high-school level, alternative schools frequently involve their students even more directly in the educational process. Whether the school is completely outside the traditional institutionalized school system or, as in some communities, alternatives are offered within the system, students take complete charge of their own learning. Beyond making choices within the classroom, among learning materials provided by a teacher, alternative-school students often decide what they will learn and how they will go about learning it.

Alternative-school students, for instance, frequently get involved in community projects. They may work to register voters or to clean up a playground. They will sometimes, even for formal academic subjects, take the responsibility for finding their own teachers. A school system may supply core teachers and an administrator. Then, if students want to learn something else, they find the teachers and set up a mutually agreeable time for the class. In one suburban school system students found an economist from a nearby university who was able to meet with interested students on a regular basis. They also found a Lufthansa stewardess willing to teach German, on a schedule built around her hours on the ground.

What do these schools have in common? They are based on the fundamental humanist belief that significant learning involves the whole person, feelings as well as thoughts. They are based on the belief that significant learning, as contrasted to the meaningless rote memorization that too often takes place in traditional classrooms, is self-initiated. They are based on the belief that what is important is the *process* of learning. Facts become out-of-date. Memorizing facts won't help when the facts change. The world is changing, humanist educators point out, and the best way to equip students to deal with a changing world is to teach them to learn for themselves. "The only man who is educated," Carl Rogers wrote in *Freedom to Learn*, "is the man who has learned how to learn."

Humanistically oriented schools are based on a number of assumptions about the process of learning: Children are innately curious; given the chance, they will explore their environment. Exploratory behavior is intrinsically rewarding and self-perpetuating; children will continue to explore their environment and to learn from it if they do not feel threatened. Confidence in the self is essential before self-directed learning can take place, before you can feel free to make choices about learning. Involvement, above all, signifies learning. Whatever absorbs your attention and your interests, even if it looks like play, is actually learning. The small child building a block tower may be "playing," but he is also learning something about the principle of gravity. The older student working street corners in a voter-registration drive may be "getting out of school," but he is also learning something about democratic government at the grass-roots level.

Humanists cite many specific examples:

• When you want to learn something, you learn it. You don't let obstacles stand in the way. Try to feed a toddler determined to snatch the spoon and master the art of feeding herself. Try not to answer the persistent "Why is grass green?" questions of a preschooler. Try to stop an adolescent who wants to learn to drive.

• When you take part in the learning process, participate rather than observe, you learn still more. Watch a chemistry experiment or perform a chemistry experiment—which is more effective? Listen to a book review or write one yourself—which is more memorable? Memorize a list of dates or seek the reasons for a historical event—which again?

• When you are treated with respect, free from the threat of insults to your self, your positive self-image allows you to concentrate on learning. Laugh at the reading errors of a third-grader and he isn't likely to volunteer to read aloud again. Snicker at the arithmetic mistake your classmate makes while doing an algebra problem at the board and he probably won't think too well of math or of you or of himself. It's bad enough when you laugh at a classmate's errors. It's worse when a teacher is mocking or sarcastic.

Compare the humanist view to the behaviorist view, as they might show up in the classroom. Humanists, in general, look at the whole child. They are concerned at least as much with social and emotional development, with communication skills and self-fulfillment, as with the purely academic. They are more interested in the process of learning than in the content. Behaviorists, on the other hand, tend to focus on competence, and to develop competence through the reinforcement of skills on a step-by-step basis. The teacher, not the student, is in charge.

These are black-and-white extremes of position. Few teachers, of course, take either extreme; most fall somewhere in between on the value continuum. But there are also small differences, differences in technique which reflect differences in philosophy. If a student acts up in class, for instance, what does the teacher do? The teacher taking the humanist orientation might try to find out what is troubling the child. This teacher might even offer personal support, by standing close to the child or placing a hand on his shoulder. The teacher following a behaviorist view would believe that attention or sympathy only provides reinforcement for the acting-out behavior. This teacher would be more likely to ignore the behavior, while praising any behavior worthy of praise, in the hope of substituting one behavior for the other.

There are other visible differences. In traditional classrooms, whether or not the teacher is following behaviorist psychology, children are seldom allowed to talk. Any verbal interplay takes place, for the most part, between an individual student and the teacher. In the open classroom, however, where students are treated as resources for one another, talk among children is encouraged. In traditional classes competitiveness among children is the rule. In humanistically based classes, where sharing is encouraged, cooperation is more often the case. In traditional classrooms, the teacher sets out to motivate the students to learn a set curriculum; the behaviorist teacher dispenses grades and gold stars much the way the behaviorist in the laboratory dispenses pellets of food to a pigeon. In open classrooms, students are expected to be self-motivated, to guide their own learning in areas which are meaningful to them.

Is one approach better than the other? That depends on your point of view. As is so often the case, research studies can be cited on both sides of the fence. But open schools and the humanist approach have been subject to increasing criticism since the days when they seemed the answer to everything that was wrong with American education. They have been accused of too much permissiveness, too much freedom, too little learning. They have been blamed for the poorer test performance of many American children in recent years. The educational pendulum is swinging, as it so often does, and the current cry is "Back to the basics," to an emphasis on reading and writing and arithmetic, to the basic academic skills.

But, many people will argue, let's not throw out the baby with the bathwater, discard everything that is good in the humanist approach along with the things that have not worked. Some children thrive in an open setting, with the opportunity to explore on their own. Others need both structure and instruction. All children, however, need to learn how to learn. Every individual, whatever the classroom orientation, benefits from being regarded as three-dimensional, as a person with feelings as well as thoughts. Every human being, child or adult, at home or at school, should be treated with respect.

PART VI

Contemporary Psychological Research

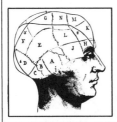

Where are we now?

Freudian psychology had, and has, an impact on the way we view ourselves. So did, and does, behaviorism. And so, too, humanism. Are you confused? How can three such different assessments of human nature all be accurate? How can they be accepted?

True, they are different. Yet each approach has a distinct contribution to make to the way in which we understand human functioning, human development, human psychology. Freud and the psychoanalytic movement made us aware of the realm of the unconscious and the importance of childhood experiences. The behaviorists have pointed up the importance of the outer world and its impact on human behavior. And the humanists emphasize the whole person, the integrated personality.

But psychology is not limited to these global views of

human personality. Much as Piaget has studied thought processes, other psychologists also work in more narrowly defined areas, seeking answers to questions about how we learn, remember, see, and react to experience. They study human beings awake and asleep, alone and in groups, at every age and stage of development. Their work has no end, because the more we know about human beings, the more we want to know.

It's impossible in a single volume to do justice to all the areas of knowledge enhanced by psychological research. It's impossible to even skim the surface. So, just as an example, this chapter will touch on some of the specific research on how people interact with people. Then, also as an example, both chapter and book will conclude with a look at a major subject of ongoing research: the subject of psychological development throughout the life cycle.

Human relationships

The ways in which we relate to other people have been extensively studied by psychologists. Human relationships encompass a wide range of psychological interaction; we will look at some elements of relationships with parents, and of relationships with other people.

Relationships with parents come first, across the animal kingdom. The earliest experiences, in infancy, determine future relationships. One of the most startling findings along these lines was made by Konrad Lorenz, who described the process of imprinting. Baby geese, Lorenz found, would follow and become attached to the first moving object they saw after they hatched. When that moving object was the mother, the goslings developed into normal geese. When the moving object was Lorenz, however, the goslings became attached to him, followed him everywhere, and, when they matured, courted human beings instead of geese.

No human has, so far as we know, been imprinted on a

goose. But the process of mother-infant bonding is undeniably important. Most hospitals today keep mothers and newborns together as much as possible instead of separating them. If they are separated, as is sometimes necessary with infants who need intensive medical care, attachment can take longer to form. And attachment is essential for normal development.

We know that attachment is essential for normal development because of psychologists' observations of the development of institutionalized children in the days when institutionalization meant mass care by indifferent caretakers. We know it, too, because psychologists have observed infant monkeys under experimental conditions.

There are a lot of similarities between infant monkeys and infant humans; one of the similarities is the need for a mother to whom the infant can cling. Harry Harlow demonstrated, in his experiments with rhesus monkeys in the early 1960s, that these monkeys, given the choice of two artificial "mothers" equipped with identical nursing bottles, one built out of wire mesh and the other out of terry cloth, would invariably choose the soft and cuddly terry-cloth form. The simple presence of the cloth form reassured the babies sufficiently so that they would explore an unfamiliar room; without the "mother" present they retreated to a corner and cried. These cloth forms became the object of attachment for the monkeys.

Live mothers and mutual attachment, of course, are better still. Both monkeys and humans are more likely to develop into psychologically normal adults, able to relate to other adults of the same species, if they have had the opportunity to form an attachment in infancy. This attachment, by the way, does not necessarily have to be with the mother. It can be with the father, a grandparent, or any caring adult. Repeated studies have shown that children do not suffer if their mothers go to work, as long as a single devoted caretaker is on hand.

Relationships with other people are studied by social psychologists. They examine the foundations of friendship, investigate racial prejudice, and consider what happens to people living in crowded cities. They look, for instance, at the degree of conformity or individuality which people exhibit in groups. Teenagers are often accused of eagerness to conform, of willingly giving in to peer pressure. Does this accusation have any foundation in fact?

A desire to conform, to blend with the crowd, it turns out, does play a significant role in human behavior. College students, frequently studied by psychologists because they are so accessible, have been volunteer subjects in many experiments. Some such experiments deal, on the surface, with perception.

In one well-known experiment by Solomon E. Asch, groups of seven students were presented with a diagram showing lines of clearly different lengths. They were asked which line was longest. Six students in each group were coached to give a wrong answer, to agree that a shorter line was longer, while the seventh student, uncoached, was giving his honest opinion. Honesty was short-lived. The seventh student (the actual subject in this experiment), thinking all seven were describing what they saw, eventually gave in to the group pressure of the wrong answer, denying the evidence he could clearly see. In some cases, of course, an independent student stuck to his own opinion. But many, far more than the researchers had expected, bent to the majority opinion.

In variations on this experiment, Asch found that disagreement by a single individual would not sway the subject. If two or more people disagreed, however, more and more subjects found it hard to trust their own judgment. If, on the other hand, just one other person in a group situation supported the subject's opinion, the subject found it possible to withstand disagreement by the majority. Also, and not surprisingly, the subject developed warm feelings toward his supporter. Does this finding ring a familiar note? Have you ever given in to your friends just because they all agreed and you were the lone dissenter? Have you ever formed a friendship on the basis of support for an unpopular position?

Other experiments on conformity also produce disturbing results. Stanley Milgram's controversial studies at Yale in the 1960s dealt with obedience. How far, he wondered, would people go to follow orders? How far would they go when they thought that, by following the orders, they were responsible for severe pain felt by another human being? Milgram set up experiments in which a subject thought that he was administering electric shocks of increasing severity to the experiment's ostensible subject. Actually, the person being "shocked" was in on the experiment and there were no shocks. But the subject did not know this. Each subject believed that more and harsher shocks were being administered, and that the pain was real. Yet most subjects continued. Most subjects apparently believed that their first obligation was to the researcher; most felt that they had to follow his orders. This kind of psychological research seems to explain, if not exonerate, what happened in Germany during World War II: Most Germans, as individuals, would have abhorred the things they were asked to do. But most Germans, like most of Milgram's subjects, thought following orders was more important.

Not all psychological experiments are performed by psychologists. Teachers sometimes set up experimental situations in order to make a point. In one recent instance, a junior-high-school teacher in California told his class that a team of Chinese gymnasts was to visit the school. The teacher asked for volunteers to show the Chinese around. Then, as the school's leading gymnast eagerly volunteered, the teacher mentioned, ever so casually, that the Chinese disliked blonds. To reinforce goodwill between the two groups, therefore, the teachers had agreed that no blond students could participate. In fact, all blonds—including the star gymnast—would have to be kept out of sight. "The horrifying thing," says the student who reported the experiment, "is that only three of us protested what was being done to our classmates. Everyone else went along. It was just like Nazi Germany."

Such experiments, although they involve manipulation (and have been questioned on ethical grounds), indicate the extent to which behavior can be swayed in ordinary circumstances by the compelling need to be accepted. We all need to be accepted, to feel secure. So we conform, to greater or lesser degree, to the expectations of our parents, our friends, our culture, our society. But we don't necessarily continue to conform. As we mature, as we develop a surer sense of self, and as we see social issues in a different light, we may feel freer to stand alone.

One thing psychologists have made abundantly clear is that personality is not fixed at any given time. People continue to grow and to change. We will conclude this brief look at psychology, therefore, with a glimpse of the ongoing research into adult development.

Life-cycle development

People used to assume, by and large, that mental and physical and emotional development was essentially a task confined to the years of childhood and adolescence. Growth and change in the first twenty years of life is clear to even the casual eye. And Freud, after all, emphasized the significance of childhood events in the psychological life of the adult. It's little wonder that developmental psychologists, until relatively recently, concentrated their attention and their research efforts on the years of childhood.

Erik H. Erikson was one of the first to go beyond childhood, to view development as a lifelong phenomenon. Erikson, a psychoanalyst who was described in Part II, speaks of "eight stages of man," eight stages of human development. The stages, in a progression from infancy through old age, are described in terms of the ego qualities which emerge in the eight critical periods of development. Each period is described in terms of a conflict between a negative and a positive outcome.

The first four stages deal with childhood, the next two with adolescence and young adulthood, and the last two with the mature individual. Stage 7, which Erikson calls Generativity vs. Stagnation, revolves around the productivity and creativity which must characterize the life of the mature adult if stagnation is not to result. That productivity may show itself in guiding the next generation; it may show itself in career-related endeavors. But it is essential for this developmental stage to occur.

Stage 8, called Ego integrity vs. Despair, characterizes the last stage of life. The mature adult who has worked through the previous stages will possess the integrity to defend his own chosen style of life. Because he is satisfied with his life as it has been lived, he can accept the likelihood of death. The individual who is not satisfied, who does not possess what Erikson calls ego integrity, despairs when death is on the horizon, because life is too short to start again.

Erikson is not suggesting that life is a series of crises. But he does believe that psychosocial development throughout the life cycle proceeds by a series of critical steps, of turning points, of moments of decision.

This thesis is being supported and extended by considerable research, as psychologists and psychiatrists on both coasts simultaneously investigate the course of adult development. The results of their research to date have recently been published in several books: Daniel J. Levinson and his co-workers at Yale have written *The Seasons of a Man's Life,* based on a study of forty men, ages thirty-five to forty-five. The forty men were divided equally among hourly blue-collar workers, executives, academic biologists, and novelists. They came from a variety of ethnic and socioeconomic backgrounds. Roger Gould at the University of California in Los Angeles has written *Transformations: Growth and Change in Adult Life,* based on hundreds of psychiatric interviews and case histories. George E. Vaillant of Harvard Medical School has written *Adaptation to Life,* the report of almost forty years of study of a group of ninety-five white male college graduates. Although it is primarily a study of mental health, Vaillant's book also deals with life-cycle development. And journalist Gail Sheehy has pulled much of this research together, and reported on her own extensive interviews with men and women, in her best-selling book, *Passages: Predictable Crises of Adult Life.*

The overall unifying theme of the research, and of the books, is that development continues throughout life. A specific theme is that development is cyclical, that people go through what Levinson calls stable periods and transitions, each of which can last for several years. And another point is that the cycles are age-related but not age-determined. People face the transition from young adulthood to midlife just as they face the transition from childhood to adolescence, within a framework of a few years but not at a specific age or because of a particular event. Marriage does not define adulthood. Retirement does not define old age. The significant events are internal.

People also face transition and change in terms of their individual personalities and the social circumstances in which they live. Development is orderly, the researchers conclude, but not necessarily predictable. The sequence is the same. The ways in which people move through the sequence, and the ways in which they react to significant external events, are different. We may now know that adults, like children, go through certain stages of development. We do not know exactly when those stages will occur or how the individual will react.

Major transitional periods seem to occur in the late teens (the "early adult transition"), at about age forty (the "mid-life transition"), and again at about age sixty (the "late adult transition"). You, in your teens, are approaching early adulthood, what Levinson calls "the most dramatic of all eras." This is the era in which a tentative and preliminary adult identity is established through basic choices of occupation and life-style. This era, this transitional phase, extends over several years, beginning and ending at different times in different people. It is an easy transition for some people, a difficult one for others. Sooner or later, however, according to the Levinson theory, every individual must face at least one developmental struggle. That struggle may occur in early adulthood; it may come much later.

Some young people begin the transition to adolescence at eleven, others at fourteen. Some breeze through adolescence without emotional turmoil, while others suffer a great deal. You may begin to make early adult choices at seventeen, while a classmate's transition begins at twenty. You may find the choice of career a straightforward and simple decision, stemming logically from earlier interests; your friend may waver among several possibilities before making a decision.

Some adults, similarly, begin what Levinson calls the mid-life transition at thirty-nine, others at forty-two. Many middle-aged adults continue to find satisfaction in their lives, in their marriages and their careers. Others, the people Vail-

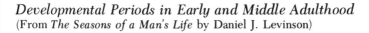

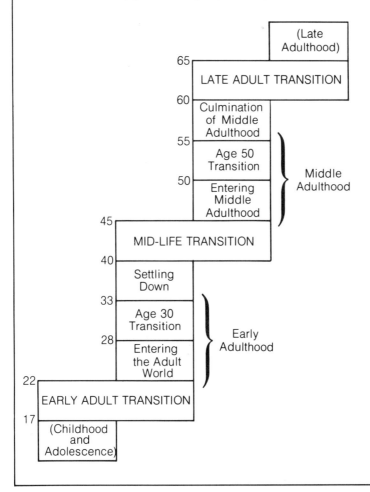

lant calls "middle-aged adolescents," begin to reorder their lives, a process which can be tumultuous both to the people themselves and to those around them. A long-lasting marriage may be dissolved, or a seemingly satisfying career may be given up in favor of another. Some observers call this the mid-life crisis. Others say that no transition is actually a crisis when it comes at the appropriate time of life.

Either way, crisis or not, perspective shifts. "The world," Vaillant notes, "looks different to the same person at different ages." Think about this when you complain that your parents don't remember what it was like to be fifteen. They may not indeed, but not because they don't want to. The same man who resisted U.S. entry into World War II could not understand his son's objections to Vietnam. The man who loved modern jazz when he was an adolescent has nothing but contempt, now that he is fifty, for his daughter's passion for rock and roll. It's more than a failure of memory. "By the time the young communist has grown into an old reactionary," Vaillant says, "the changes within have been so imperceptible, if so profound, that he believes that he still sees with the same eyes and feels with the same heart. He believes that only the times have changed."

These studies of adult development are only a beginning. They do not, for the most part, deal with women. Most psychologists believe that women go through similar life-cycle development but, perhaps, at a different pace. Sheehy concluded, after her interviews, that men and women are developmentally "out of sync," traveling along different paths, for much of adult life. Levinson and his co-workers at Yale are just beginning a long-range study of women which should provide more information.

These studies also do not deal with development much beyond the late forties. Most people who work with older adults believe nonetheless that development and growth and change and adaptability continue to the very end of life. This has been suggested in Erik Erikson's work. And it has been strongly indicated by Dr. Robert N. Butler and his colleagues at the National Institute of Aging, although not in specific terms of critical periods. This, too, remains to be documented.

There is little doubt, meanwhile, that new knowledge of adult development means new understanding of human personality. This new understanding can help you. When you ask your parents to remember, for instance, that you are "going through a stage," you might remember that they are too. When you look ahead to your own life, you needn't think that it will all be over at thirty. Adults are not on some emotional plateau, immune to change. Your parents, and you, will continue to grow.

BIBLIOGRAPHY
*Recommended

GENERAL READINGS

*Beekman, Daniel. *The Mechanical Baby: A Popular History of the Theory and Practice of Child Raising.* Westport, Conn.: Lawrence Hill & Company Publishers, 1977.

Buhler, Charlotte. *Psychology for Contemporary Living.* New York: Hawthorn Books, 1968.

*Cable, Mary. *The Little Darlings. A History of Child Rearing in America.* New York: Charles Scribner's Sons, 1972, 1974, 1975.

*Cohen, David, ed. *Psychologists on Psychology.* New York: Taplinger Publishing Co., 1976.

*Hall, Elizabeth. *Why We Do What We Do.* Boston: Houghton Mifflin Company, 1973.

Rosenbaum, Jean. *Is Your Volkswagen a Sex Symbol? What Your Life-Style Reveals About You and Your Personality.* New York: Hawthorn Books, 1972.

Sargent, S. Stansfeld, and Stafford, Kenneth R. *Basic Teachings of the Great Psychologists.* Garden City, N.Y.: Doubleday & Co., Dolphin Books, 1944, 1965.

Skolnick, Arlene. "The Myth of the Vulnerable Child." *Psychology Today,* Fall 1978, pp. 56–65.

Spock, Benjamin. *Baby and Child Care.* New York: Pocket Books, Inc., 1957.

———. *Raising Children in a Difficult Time.* New York: W. W. Norton & Co., 1974.

PART I

Asimov, Isaac. *Words From the Myths.* Boston: Houghton Mifflin Company, 1961.

Bulfinch, Thomas. *Bulfinch's Mythology.* New York: Collier Books, 1962.

Davidoff, Linda L. *Introduction to Psychology.* New York: McGraw-Hill, 1976.

*Field, D. M. *Greek and Roman Mythology.* New York: Chartwell Books, 1977.

PART II

*Bettelheim, Bruno. *The Uses of Enchantment.* New York: Alfred A. Knopf, 1976.

Brim, Orville G., Jr. *Education for Child Rearing.* New York: Free Press, 1959, 1965.

Cheskin, Louis. *Why People Buy.* New York: Liveright, 1959.

Chesler, Phyllis. *Women & Madness*. Garden City, N.Y.: Doubleday & Co., 1972.

Chess, Dr. Stella. "Can I blame my parents for who I am?" *The Record*, Hackensack, N.J., July 12, 1978.

Dichter, Ernest. *The Strategy of Desire*. Garden City, N.Y.: Doubleday & Co., 1960.

Erikson, Erik H. *Childhood and Society*. New York: W. W. Norton & Co., 1950, 1963.

Ewen, Stuart. *Captains of Consciousness: Advertising and the Social Roots of the Consumer Culture*. New York: McGraw-Hill Book Company, 1976.

Fodor, Nandor, and Gaynor, Frank, eds. *Freud: Dictionary of Psychoanalysis*. Greenwich, Conn.: Fawcett Publications, Inc., 1958.

*Fraiberg, Selma. *The Magic Years*. New York: Charles Scribner's Sons, 1959.

Freeman, Lucy, ed. *Celebrities On the Couch*. Los Angeles: Price/Stern/Sloan Publishers, n.d.

Freud, Sigmund. *The Ego and the Id*. Translated by Joan Riviere, edited by James Strachey. New York: W. W. Norton & Co., 1960.

*———. *A General Introduction to Psychoanalysis*. New York: Pocket Books, 1963.

Goldstein, Joseph; Freud, Anna; and Solnit, Albert J. *Beyond the Best Interests of the Child*. New York: Free Press, 1973.

Gross, Martin L. *The Brain Watchers*. New York: Random House, 1962.

*———. *The Psychological Society*. New York: Random House, 1978. (A critical look.)

Grotjahn, Martin. *Psychoanalysis and the Family Neurosis*. New York: W. W. Norton & Co., 1960.

Jung, C. G., The Basic Writings of Edited by Violet deLaszlo. New York: Random House, Modern Library, 1959.

*Kardiner, A. *My Analysis With Freud: Reminiscences*. New York: W. W. Norton & Co., 1977.

Lear, Martha Weinman. "Daddies." *The New York Times*, June 18, 1978.

Mead, Margaret. *Male and Female*. New York: Wm. F. Morrow, 1949.

Roazen, Paul. *Erik H. Erikson*. New York: Free Press, 1976.

*———. *Freud and His Followers*. New York: Alfred A. Knopf, 1975.

Stoutenberg, Adrien, and Baker, Laura Nelson. *Explorer of the Unconscious: Sigmund Freud*. New York: Charles Scribner's Sons, 1965.

Strouse, Jean, ed. *Women & Analysis*. New York: Grossman Publishers, Viking Press, 1974.

Thomas, Alexander; Chess, Stella; Birch, Herbert G.; Hertzig, Margaret E.; and Korn, Sam. *Behavioral Individuality in Early Childhood*. New York: New York University Press, 1963.

Wollheim, Richard. *Sigmund Freud*. New York: Viking Press, 1971.

PART III

Bry, Adelaide. *A Primer of Behavioral Psychology*. New York: New American Library, Mentor Books, 1975.

*Fensterheim, Herbert, and Baer, Jean. *Don't Say Yes When You Want To Say No*. New York: David McKay Co., 1975.

Gray, F.; Grawbard, P. S.; and Rosenberg, H. "Little Brother Is Changing You." *Psychology Today*, March 1974, pp. 42–46.

*Huxley, Aldous. *Brave New World*. New York: Harper & Row, 1932, 1946.

————. *Brave New World Revisited*. New York: Harper & Row, 1958.

Lefrancois, Guy R. *Psychology for Teaching: A Bear Always Faces the Front*. Belmont, Calif.: Wadsworth Publishing Co., 1972.

"Psychology Clinic for Disturbed Pets Sometimes Puts the Owners on the Couch." *The New York Times*, April 22, 1978.

*Robbins, Jhan, and Fisher, Dave. *How to Make and Break Habits*. New York: Dell Publishing Co., Inc. 1973.

*Schrag, Peter. *Mind Control*. New York: Pantheon Books, 1978.

*Skinner, B. F. *About Behaviorism*. New York: Alfred A. Knopf, 1974.

*————. *Walden Two*. New York: Macmillan, 1948, 1976.

————. "Why Don't We Use the Behavioral Sciences?" *Human Nature*, March 1978, pp. 86–92.

"Skinner's Utopia: Panacea, or Path to Hell?" *Time*, September 20, 1971.

Smith, Wendell I., and Moore, J. William. *Conditioning and Instrumental Learning*. New York: McGraw-Hill, 1966.

Snortum, John R. "Self-Modification: Ben Franklin's Pursuit of Perfection." *Psychology Today*, April 1976, pp. 80–83.

Stern, Frances Merritt, and Hoch, Ruth S.; with Carper, Jean. *Mind Trips To Help You Lose Weight*. Chicago: Playboy Press, 1976.

Watson, John B. "Psychology as the Behaviorist Views It." 1913. In *Readings in the History of Psychology*, edited by Wayne Dennis. New York: Appleton-Century-Crofts, 1948.

Wesley, Frank. *Childrearing Psychology*. New York: Behavioral Publications, 1971.

PART IV

*Beadle, Muriel. *A Child's Mind*. Garden City, N.Y.: Doubleday & Co., Anchor Books, 1970.

Brearly, Molly. *The Teaching of Young Children*. New York: Schocken Books, 1970.

Ginsburg, Herbert, and Opper, Sylvia. *Piaget's Theory of Intellectual Development*. Englewood Cliffs, N.J.: Prentice-Hall, 1969.

Muss, Rolf E. *Theories of Adolescence*. New York: Random House, 1962, 1968.

Pulaski, Mary Ann Spencer. *Understanding Piaget*. New York: Harper & Row, 1971.

Renner, John W.; Stafford, Donald G.; Lawson, Anton E.; McKinnon, Joe W.; Friot, F. Elizabeth; and Kellogg, Donald H. *Research, Teaching, and Learning with the Piaget Model*. Norman, Okla.: University of Oklahoma Press, 1976.

Wadsworth, Barry J. *Piaget's Theory of Cognitive Development*. New York: David McKay Co., 1971.

PART V

Featherstone, Joseph. *Schools Where Children Learn*. New York: Avon Books, Discus, 1971.

Hamachek, Don E. *Behavior Dynamics in Teaching, Learning, and Growth*. Boston: Allyn & Bacon, 1975.

Havemann, Ernest. "Alternatives to Analysis." *Annual Editions Readings in Psychology '72–'73*. Guilford, Conn.: Dushkin Publishing Group, 1973.

Maslow, A. H. "Self-Actualizing People." In *Symposia on Topical Issues*, edited by W. Wolff, vol. I, "Values in Personality Research," pp. 11–34. New York: Grune & Stratton, 1950.

———. *Toward a Psychology of Being*. New York: D. Van Nostrand Company, 1968.

Mishara, Brian L., and Patterson, Robert D. *Consumer's Guide to Mental Health*. New York: Times Books, 1977.

Rathbone, Charles H., ed. *Open Education: The Informal Classroom*. New York: Scholastic Book Services, Citation Press, 1971.

Raths, Louis E.; Harmin, Merrill; and Simon, Sidney B. *Values and Teaching*. Columbus, Ohio: Charles E. Merrill Publishing Company, 1966.

Rogers, Carl. *Carl Rogers on Encounter Groups*. New York: Harper & Row, 1970.

———. *Carl Rogers On Personal Power*. New York: Delacorte Press, 1977.

———. *Freedom to Learn: A View of What Education Might Become*. Columbus, Ohio: Charles E. Merrill Publishing Company, 1969.

———. *On Becoming a Person*. Boston: Houghton Mifflin Company, 1961.

———. "Personal Power At Work." *Psychology Today*, April 1977, pp. 60–62, 93–94.

Silberman, Charles E. *Crisis in the Classroom*. New York: Random House, 1970.

*Simon, Sidney B. *Meeting Yourself Halfway*. Niles, Ill.: Argus Communications, 1974. (Thirty-one values-clarification strategies for daily living.)

Valett, Robert. *Self-Actualization*. Niles, Ill.: Argus Communications, 1974.

Yelon, Stephen L., and Weinstein, Grace W. *A Teacher's World: Psychology in the Classroom*. McGraw-Hill, 1977.

PART VI

Bower, Gordon H. "Improving Memory." *Human Nature*, February 1978, pp. 64–72.

Erikson, Erik H. *Childhood and Society*. New York: W. W. Norton & Co., 1963.

Frontiers of Psychological Research. San Francisco: W. H. Freeman & Company Publishers, 1966. (Readings from *Scientific American*.)

Gould, Roger L. *Transformations: Growth and Change in Adult Life*. New York: Simon & Schuster, 1978.

*Levinson, Daniel J., with Darrow, Charlotte N.; Klein, Edward B.; Levinson, Maria H.; and McKee, Braxton. *The Seasons of a Man's Life*. New York: Alfred A. Knopf, 1978.

*Sheehy, Gail. *Passages: Predictable Crises of Adult Life*. New York: E. P. Dutton & Co., 1974, 1976.

*Vaillant, George E. *Adaptation to Life*. Boston: Little, Brown & Company, 1977.

INDEX

imprinting, 117
individual psychology (Adler), 25
Individually Prescribed Instruction
    (IPI), 69–70
inferiority complex, 25
instinct theories, 14, 26
    sexual, 16, 17, 21, 23, 25, 26
    unconscious and, 19, 22, 35
intelligence, 78
    IQ and, 12, 90

Jones, Mary Cover, 49
Jung, Carl Gustav, 25–26

Lear, Martha Weinman, 18
Lefrancois, Guy, 56
Levinson, Daniel J., 123, 124, 126
libido, 16, 22, 23, 25, 26
life-cycle development, 16–17, 27–
    28, 121–127
"little Albert" case, 48–49
Lorenz, Konrad, 117
love, demonstrations of, 64–65

Maslow, Abraham, 91, 92–94, 101
"me" society, 99–100
Mead, Margaret, 64
Milgram, Stanley, 120
models (Maslow), 92
mutual problem solving (Gordon),
    106–107
myths and fairy tales, 8–11

narcissism, 9–10
neuroses, 26, 32
    discussion of, 4–5
    Freudian concepts of, 16, 19–21,
        31, 43
    humanistic view of, 98
normality, 16
    definition of, 5–6
    expectations and, 5–8
    Freudian view of, 43
    humanism and, 91

object permanence (Piaget), 80–81
Oedipus complex, 10, 17–18, 32,
    37–38, 42
Oedipus myth, 9, 10, 17
open education, 110–111
operant conditioning, 45, 46, 47,
    50–58, 65–75
oral stage, 16, 31, 80

paranoia, 4
parent-child interaction, 36–39,
    62–66, 102–107, 117–119
Parent Effectiveness Training
    (P.E.T.), 104–107
Pavlov's experiments, 46, 52
peak experiences (Maslow), 93, 94
penis envy, 17, 42–44
permissiveness, 36, 61, 115
personality theories
    behavioristic, 45, 47–48, 50,
        57–58
    humanistic, 89–115
    psychoanalytic, 10, 14, 16–29, 32,
        35–42
phallic stage, 16, 17
phobias, 4–5, 20
Piaget, Jean, 13, 76–88, 117
pleasure principle, 19, 31
programmed instruction, 68–70
psyche, 2–3, 4
Psyche legend, 2–3
psychiatry, 3
psychoanalytic theory, 13, 14–44,
    90–91
    behaviorism vs., 45, 47, 49, 54,
        65, 75
    childhood development and,
        16–20, 26–27, 31, 35–42, 65
    critics of, 31–32, 39–44
    influences of, 14, 30–31, 33–38,
        42–44, 65, 78, 116
    successors to Freud in, 24–29
    therapy and, 15, 18–19, 22–25,
        31–33